T0221002

Praise for
News & Numbers

"*News & Numbers* is a classic that should be a must-read for journalists in all fields, from business to sports. It provides practical advice for avoiding embarrassing statistical pitfalls."

Cristine Russell, President, Council for the Advancement of Science Writing

"The demand for press coverage of science and medicine is growing as public interest grows. This book sets the standard. It uses simple language to teach the layman or the scientist how to read and understand scientific publications. Even more important, it teaches one to critically interpret and think about research findings and ask the right questions. This is a book that you can read from cover to cover and then keep as a reference."

Otis Brawley, Chief Medical and Scientific Officer, American Cancer Society

"Vic Cohn's reporting inspired a generation of science and health writers, and he kept us on the straight and narrow with his concise and engaging book on how to interpret scientific studies. Now updated and expanded, his classic guide to statistics should be essential reading, not just for reporters but for anybody trying to separate science from pseudoscience in the torrent of unfiltered information flowing over the internet."

Colin Norman, News Editor, *Science* magazine

"The third edition of *News & Numbers* is welcomed, bringing alive again with new examples the wisdom and uncommon common sense of a great man and missed colleague. The updates by Lewis Cope and Vic's daughter, Deborah Cohn Runkle, add freshness and immediacy to the advice Vic gave."

Fritz Scheuren, 100th President, American Statistical Association

Third
Edition

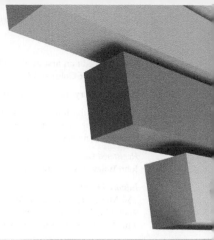

NEWS & NUMBERS
A WRITER'S GUIDE TO STATISTICS

Victor Cohn and
Lewis Cope

with Deborah Cohn Runkle

WILEY-BLACKWELL

A John Wiley & Sons, Ltd., Publication

This third edition first published 2012
© 2012 Victor Cohn and Lewis Cope

Edition history: 1e 1989; Blackwell Publishing Professional (2e, 2001)

Blackwell Publishing was acquired by John Wiley & Sons in February 2007. Blackwell's
publishing program has been merged with Wiley's global Scientific, Technical, and Medical
business to form Wiley-Blackwell.

Registered Office
John Wiley & Sons Ltd, The Atrium, Southern Gate, Chichester, West Sussex, PO19 8SQ, UK

Editorial Offices
350 Main Street, Malden, MA 02148-5020, USA
9600 Garsington Road, Oxford, OX4 2DQ, UK
The Atrium, Southern Gate, Chichester, West Sussex, PO19 8SQ, UK

For details of our global editorial offices, for customer services, and for information about how
to apply for permission to reuse the copyright material in this book please see our website at
www.wiley.com/wiley-blackwell.

The right of Victor Cohn and Lewis Cope to be identified as the authors of this work has been
asserted in accordance with the UK Copyright, Designs and Patents Act 1988.

All rights reserved. No part of this publication may be reproduced, stored in a retrieval system,
or transmitted, in any form or by any means, electronic, mechanical, photocopying, recording
or otherwise, except as permitted by the UK Copyright, Designs and Patents Act 1988,
without the prior permission of the publisher.

Wiley also publishes its books in a variety of electronic formats. Some content that appears in
print may not be available in electronic books.

Designations used by companies to distinguish their products are often claimed as trademarks.
All brand names and product names used in this book are trade names, service marks,
trademarks or registered trademarks of their respective owners. The publisher is not associated
with any product or vendor mentioned in this book. This publication is designed to provide
accurate and authoritative information in regard to the subject matter covered. It is sold
on the understanding that the publisher is not engaged in rendering professional services.
If professional advice or other expert assistance is required, the services of a competent
professional should be sought.

Library of Congress Cataloging-in-Publication Data

Cohn, Victor, 1919–2000
    News & numbers : a writer's guide to statistics / Victor Cohn, Lewis Cope.—3rd ed. / with
Deborah Cohn Runkle.
        p.   cm.
    Includes bibliographical references and index.
    ISBN 978-1-4443-6188-9 (hardcover : alk. paper)—ISBN 978-1-4051-6096-4 (pbk.)
1. Public health—Statistics.   2. Environmental health—Statistics.   3. Vital statistics.
I. Cope, Lewis, 1934–   II. Cohn Runkle, Deborah.   III. Title.   IV. Title: News
and numbers.
    RA407.C64 2011
    614.4′20727–dc23
                                            2011017059
A catalogue record for this book is available from the British Library.

This book is published in the following electronic formats: ePDFs 9781444344332;
epub 9781444344349; Kindle 9781444344356.

Set in 10/12.5pt Plantin by SPi Publisher Services, Pondicherry, India

1   2012

Contents

Contents

A Note to Our Readers

This is a book to help you decide which numbers and studies you probably can trust and which ones you surely should trash.

The rules of statistics are the rules of clear thinking, codified. This book explains the role, logic, and language of statistics, so that we can ask better questions and get better answers.

While the book's largest audience has been health and other science writers, we believe that it can also be helpful to many other writers and editors, as well as to students of journalism. Health studies are emphasized in many of the chapters because they are so important and they illustrate many principles so well. But this book shows how statistical savvy can help in writing about business, education, environmental policy, sports, opinion polls, crime, and other topics.

News & Numbers is the brainchild of the late Victor Cohn, a former science editor of the *Washington Post* and sole author of the first edition. I'm glad I could help with later editions, but this is still "Vic's book." His inspiring spirit lives on with this edition.

I am particularly pleased that one of his daughters, Deborah Cohn Runkle, a science policy analyst at the American Association for the Advancement of Science, has provided her expertise to help update and expand this latest edition of *News & Numbers*.

We've added a chapter to delve deeper into writing about risks. With President Obama's health system overhaul plan now law, we've added new things to think about in the chapter on health care costs and quality. There's also a new section on "missing numbers" in the last chapter that we hope will stir your thinking. And we've added other new information that we hope you will enjoy along with the old.

Lewis Cope

A Tribute to Victor Cohn, 1919–2000

Victor was a pioneer science writer and a master of his craft. Often referred to as the "Dean of Science Writers," he became the gold standard for others in his profession.

Beginning his career in the mid-1940s, following service as a naval officer in World War II, he quickly showed an uncanny ability to write about complex medical and other scientific topics in clear, easy-to-understand ways. He provided millions of readers with stories about the landing of the first humans on the moon, the development of the polio vaccine, the then-new field of transplant surgery, the latest trends in health care insurance and medical plans, and many, many other exciting developments over a career that lasted more than 50 years. Throughout, he remained diligent at explaining the cost and ethical issues that came with some of the advances, particularly in the medical sciences.

As part of all this, he showed his fellow journalists the importance of probing numbers to discover what they can reveal about virtually every aspect of our lives. He wrote *News & Numbers* to share his techniques for doing this in the most revealing and the most responsible way. His quest for excellence in reporting lives on in the Victor Cohn Prize for Excellence in Medical Science Writing, awarded yearly by the Council for the Advancement of Science Writing. With this new edition, Victor's message lives on.

Lewis Cope, coauthor of this edition

Foreword

I've long thought that if journalists could be sued for malpractice, many of us would have been found guilty some time ago. We often err in ways that inevitably harm the public – for example, by distorting reality, or framing issues in deceptively false terms. Among the tools we sometimes wield dangerously as we commit our version of malpractice is the subject of this book: numbers. At one time or another, most of us have written a story that either cited as evidence some number of dubious provenance, or that used numbers or statistics in ways that suggested that the meaning of a medical study or other set of findings was entirely lost upon on us.

Fortunately for many of us, before we did any serious harm, someone handed us a copy of Vic Cohn's marvelous *News & Numbers*, now released in a third edition co-authored by Vic and Lewis Cope, with the assistance of Vic's talented daughter, Deborah Cohn Runkle. I was rescued in this fashion early in my journalistic career, and later had the honor of meeting Cohn and thanking him for his wonderful book. With the advent of this new edition, it is heartening that an entirely new generation of journalists will now have the chance to be saved similarly from their sins.

Much of the content of this book will be familiar to readers of previous editions, even as some of the examples have been updated to reflect recent events, such as the now-discredited vaccines-cause-autism controversy, or the 2010 BP oil spill in the Gulf of Mexico. Perhaps the most important lesson is that almost all stories of a scientific nature deal with an element of uncertainty. And with so much to study amid the rapidly changing sciences of medicine and health care, "truth" often looks more like the images of a constantly shifting kaleidoscope than a message carved on a stone tablet. Thus the book's excellent advice: "Good reporters try to tell their readers and viewers the degree of uncertainty," using words such as "may" or "evidence indicates" and seldom words like "proof."

From the standpoint of the First Amendment, it's a good thing for society that reporters don't have to be licensed. But it's not so good that one can become a reporter – even for an esteemed national publication or news channel – without even a rudimentary grasp of statistics. This book's crash course on probability, statistical power, bias, and variability is the equivalent of educating a novice driver about the rules of the road. Readers will also be introduced to the wide array of types of medical and scientific studies, and the strengths and weaknesses of each.

Portions of several chapters are devoted to the all-important topic of writing about risk. Important concepts are defined and differentiated, such as relative risk and absolute risk – two different ways of measuring risk that should always be stated together, to give readers the broadest possible understanding of a particular harm. A useful discussion focuses not just on distortions that journalists may make, but common public perceptions and misperceptions that affect the way readers or viewers respond to various risks.

Among the new entries in this edition is a chapter on health costs, quality, and insurance, which wisely cautions careful observation of the effects of the 2010 Affordable Care Act. Because this chapter was written so far ahead of the implementation of most of the law in 2014, its main message is "wait and see" what happens. Perhaps equally important is to encourage journalists to consider and convey to our audiences the totality of the law's effects, which inevitably will bring tradeoffs – for example, possibly more spending on health care because many more Americans have health insurance. As critical as verifying the "numbers" coming out of health reform will be understanding how the many different sets of numbers will relate to each other, and what values – and I don't mean numerical ones – Americans will assign to the collective results.

Overall, this new edition upholds Cohn's perspective that behind bad use of numbers is usually bad thinking, sometimes by the user and sometimes by the person who cooked up the numbers in the first place. And Cohn was a staunch believer in the notion that journalists had a duty to be good thinkers. This edition's epilogue quotes a list Cohn once made of what constitutes a good reporter; one entry asserts, "A good reporter is privileged to contribute to the great fabric of news that democracy requires." This edition powerfully evokes Cohn's spirit, and his belief that, with that privilege, the responsibility also comes to get the facts – and the numbers – right.

Susan Dentzer
Editor-in-Chief, *Health Affairs*

Acknowledgments

Victor Cohn's main mentor and guide in preparation of the first edition of this book was Dr. Frederick Mosteller of the Harvard School of Public Health. The project was supported by the Russell Sage Foundation and by the Council for the Advancement of Science Writing.

Cohn did much of the original work as a visiting fellow at the Harvard School of Public Health, where Dr. Jay Winsten, director of the Center for Health Communications, was another indispensable guide. Drs. John Bailar III, Thomas A. Louis, and Marvin Zelen were valuable helpers, as were Drs Gary D. Friedman and Thomas M. Vogt at the Kaiser organizations; Michael Greenberg at Rutgers University; and Peter Montague of Princeton University. (For those who aided Cohn with the first edition of this book, the references generally are to their universities or other affiliations at the time of that edition's publication.)

For their assistance with later editions, special thanks go to: Dr. Michael Osterholm of the University of Minnesota, for his great help on epidemiology; Rob Daves, director of the Minnesota Poll at the Minneapolis-St. Paul *Star Tribune*, for sharing his great expertise on polling; and Dr. Margaret Wang of the University of Missouri-Columbia, for her great enthusiasm about all aspects of patient care.

Very special thanks go to Cohn's daughter Deborah Cohn Runkle, a senior program associate at the American Association for the Advancement of Science. Without her encouragement and assistance, this edition would not have been possible.

Others who provided valuable counsel for the second edition include Dr. Phyllis Wingo of the American Cancer Society; Dr. Ching Wang at Stanford University; John Ullmann, executive director of the World Press

Institute at Macalester College in St. Paul; and the great library staff at the *Star Tribune* in Minneapolis-St. Paul.

Many other people helped with the first edition of this book. Thanks go to Drs. Stuart A. Bessler, Syntex Corporation; H. Jack Geiger, City University of New York; Nicole Schupf Geiger, Manhattanville College; Arnold Relman, *New England Journal of Medicine*; Eugene Robin, Stanford University; and Sidney Wolfe, Public Citizen Health Research Group. Thanks also go to Katherine Wallman, Council of Professional Associations on Federal Statistics; Howard L. Lewis, American Heart Association; Philip Meyer, University of North Carolina; Lynn Ries, National Cancer Institute; Mildred Spencer Sanes; and Earl Ubell – and also Harvard's Drs. Peter Braun, Harvey Fineberg, Howard Frazier, Howard Hiatt, William Hsaio, Herb Sherman, and William Stason.

This book has been aided in the past by the Robert Wood Johnson Foundation, the Ester A. and Joseph Klingenstein Fund, and the American Statistical Association, with additional help from the Commonwealth Fund and Georgetown University.

Despite all this great help, any misstatements remain the authors' responsibility.

Notes on Sources

Book citations – The full citations for some frequently cited books are given in the bibliography.

Interviews and affiliations – Unless otherwise indicated, quotations from the following are from interviews: Drs. Michael Osterholm, University of Minnesota; John C. Bailar III, Peter Braun, Harvey Fineberg, Thomas A. Louis, Frederick Mosteller, and Marvin Zelen, at Harvard School of Public Health: H. Jack Geiger, City University of New York; and Arnold Relman, *New England Journal of Medicine*. In most cases, people cited throughout the book are listed with their academic affiliations at the time that they first were quoted in an edition of *News & Numbers*.

Quotations from seminars – Two other important sources for this manual were Drs. Peter Montague at Princeton University (director, Hazardous Waste Research Program) and Michael Greenberg at Rutgers University (director, Public Policy and Education Hazardous and Toxic Substances Research Center). Quotations are from their talks at symposiums titled "Public Health and the Environment: The Journalist's Dilemma," sponsored by the Council for the Advancement of Science Writing (CASW) at Syracuse University, April 1982; St. Louis, March 1983; and Ohio State University, April 1984.

Part I

Learning the Basics

A Guide to Part I of
News & Numbers

In the first five chapters, we cover the basics:

1. **Where We Can Do Better**
   Improving how stories with numbers are reported.

2. **The Certainty of Uncertainty**
   Scientists are always changing their minds.

3. **Testing the Evidence**
   Thinking clearly about scientific studies.

4. **What Makes a Good Study?**
   Separating the wheat from the chaff.

5. **Your Questions and Peer Review**
   What to ask the experts.

1

Where We Can Do Better

Almost everyone has heard that "figures don't lie, but liars can figure."
We need statistics, but liars give them a bad name, so to be able to tell the
liars from the statisticians is crucial.

Dr. Robert Hook

A team of medical researchers reports that it has developed a promising, even exciting, new treatment. Is the claim justified, or could there be some other explanation for their patients' improvement? Are there too few patients to justify *any* claim?

An environmentalist says that a certain toxic waste will cause many cases of cancer. An industry spokesman denies it. What research has been done? What are the numbers? How valid are they?

We watch the numbers fly in debates ranging from pupil-testing to global warming to the cost of health insurance reforms, and from influenza threats to shocking events such as the catastrophic Deepwater Horizon oil spill in the Gulf of Mexico in April 2010.

Even when we journalists say that we are dealing in facts and ideas, much of what we report is based on numbers. Politics comes down to votes. Dollar-figures dominate business and government news – and stir hot-button issues such as sports stadium proposals. Numbers are at the heart of crime rates, nutritional advice, unemployment reports, weather forecasts, and much more.

News & Numbers: A Writer's Guide to Statistics, Third Edition. Victor Cohn and
Lewis Cope with Deborah Cohn Runkle.
© 2012 Victor Cohn and Lewis Cope. Published 2012 by Blackwell Publishing Ltd.

But numbers offered by experts sometimes conflict, triggering confusion and controversies. Statistics are used or misused even by people who tell us, "I don't believe in statistics," then claim that all of us, or most people, or many do such and such. We should not merely repeat such numbers, but interpret them to deliver the best possible picture of reality.

And the really good news: We can do this without any heavy-lifting math. We do need to learn how the best statisticians – the best figurers – think. They can show us how to detect possible biases and bugaboos in numbers. And they can teach us how to consider alternate explanations, so that we won't be stuck with the obvious when the obvious is wrong.

Clear thinking is more important than any figuring. There's only one math equation in this book: $1 = 200,000$. This is our light-hearted way of expressing how one person in a poll can represent the views of up to 200,000 Americans. That is, when the poll is done right. The chapter on polling tells you how to know when things go wrong.

Although *News & Numbers* is written primarily to aid journalists in ferreting meaning out of numbers, this book can help anyone answer three questions about all sorts of studies and statistical claims:

What can I believe? What does it mean? How can I explain it to others?

The Journalistic Challenges

The very way in which we journalists tell our readers and viewers about a medical, environmental, or other controversy can affect the outcome.

If we ignore a bad situation, the public may suffer. If we write "danger," the public may quake. If we write "no danger," the public may be falsely reassured.

If we paint an experimental medical treatment too brightly, the public is given false hope. If we are overly critical of some drug that lots of people take, people may avoid a treatment that could help them, maybe even save their lives.

Simply using your noggin when you view the numbers can help you travel the middle road.

And whether we journalists will it or not, we have in effect become part of the regulatory apparatus. Dr. Peter Montague at Princeton University tells us: "The environmental and toxic situation is so complex, we can't possibly have enough officials to monitor it. Reporters help officials decide where to focus their activity."

And when to kick some responses into high gear. During the early days after the Deepwater Horizon oil well explosion, both company (BP) and federal officials tended to soft-pedal and underestimate the extent of the problem. Aggressive reporters found experts who sharply hiked the estimates of how much oil was pouring into the Gulf. These journalists provided running tallies of the miles of shorelines where gooey globs were coming ashore, the numbers of imperiled birds and wildlife, and the number of cleanup workers feeling ill effects. Nightly news broadcasts showed graphic video of oil gushing out of the ground a mile under the Gulf. National attention was soon galvanized on the crisis; both government and industry action intensified.

Five Areas for Improvement

As we reporters seek to make page one or the six o'clock news:

1. **We sometimes overstate and oversimplify.** We may report, "A study showed that black is white," when a study merely suggested there was some evidence that such might be the case. We may slight or omit the fact that a scientist calls a result "preliminary," rather than saying that it offers strong and convincing evidence.

   Dr. Thomas Vogt, at the Kaiser Permanente Center for Health Research, tells of seeing the headline "Heart Attacks from Lack of 'C'" and then, two months later, "People Who Take Vitamin C Increase Their Chances of a Heart Attack."[1] Both stories were based on limited, far-from-conclusive animal studies.

   Philip Meyer, veteran reporter and author of *Precision Journalism*, writes, "Journalists who misinterpret statistical data usually tend to err in the direction of over-interpretation … The reason for this professional bias is self-evident; you usually can't write a snappy lead upholding [the negative]. A story purporting to show that apple pie makes you sterile is more interesting than one that says there is no evidence that apple pie changes your life."[2]

   We've joked that there are only two types of health news stories – New Hope and No Hope. In truth, we must remember that the truth usually lies somewhere in the middle.

2. **We work fast, sometimes too fast,** with severe limits on the space or airtime we may fill. We find it hard to tell editors or news directors, "I haven't had enough time. I don't have the story yet." Even a

long-term project or special may be hurriedly done. In a newsroom, "long term" may mean a few weeks.

A major Southern newspaper had to print a front-page retraction after a series of stories alleged that people who worked at or lived near a plutonium plant suffered in excess numbers from a blood disease. "Our reporters obviously had confused statistics and scientific data," the editor admitted. "We did not ask enough questions."[3]

3. **We too often omit needed cautions and perspective.** We tend to rely too much on "authorities" who are either most quotable or quickly available or both. They may get carried away with their own sketchy, unconfirmed but "exciting" data – or have big axes to grind, however lofty their motives. The cautious, unbiased scientist who says, "Our results are inconclusive" or "We don't have enough data yet to make any strong statement" or "I don't know" tends to be omitted or buried deep down in the story.

Some scientists who overstate their results deserve part of the blame. But bad science is no excuse for bad journalism.

We may write too glowingly about some experimental drug to treat a perilous disease, without needed perspective about what hurdles lie ahead. We may over-worry our readers about *preliminary* evidence of a *possible* new carcinogen – yet not write often enough about what the U.S. surgeon general calls the "now undisputable" evidence that secondhand tobacco smoke "is a serious health hazard."[4]

4. **Seeking balance in our reporting on controversial issues, we sometimes forget to emphasize where the scientific evidence points.**

Study after study has found no evidence that childhood immunizations can cause autism – yet lay promoters (and some doctors) continue to garner ink and airtime on a popular daytime TV show (see Chapter 12).

On the hot-button issue of "global warming," we must not get carried away by occasional super-cold winters. Year-to-year temperatures vary by their very nature. Climate experts had to study decades of weather and interpret data going back thousands of years to detect the slow, yet potentially dangerous, warming of our planet. *The bottom line*: Most scientists now agree that global warming is real, and is linked to the burning of fossil fuels. The scientific and societal debate continues over details such as how urgent the threat might be – and precisely what to do about it. *Another bottom line*: Don't write the nay-sayers off as kooks and tools of industry. Sometimes even very minority views turn out to be right (see Chapter 9).

5. **We are influenced by intense competition** and other pressures to tell the story first and tell it most dramatically. One reporter said, "The fact is, you are going for the strong [lead and story]. And, while not patently absurd, it may not be the lead you would go for a year later."[5]

Or even a few hours later. Witness the competitive rush to declare election-night winners, and the mistakes that sometimes result.

We are also subject to human hope and human fear. A new "cure" comes along, and we want to believe it. A new alarm is sounded, and we too tremble – and may overstate the risk. Dr. H. Jack Geiger, a respected former science writer who became a professor of medicine, says:

I know I wrote stories in which I explained or interpreted the results wrongly. I wrote stories that didn't have the disclaimers I should have written. I wrote stories under competitive pressure, when it became clear later that I shouldn't have written them. I wrote stories when I hadn't asked – because I didn't know enough to ask – "Was your study capable of getting the answers you wanted? Could it be interpreted to say something else? Did you take into account possible confounding factors?"

How can we learn to do better? How do we separate the wheat from the chaff in all sorts of statistical claims and controversies? That's what the rest of this book is all about.

Notes

1. Vogt, *Making Health Decisions*.
2. Meyer, *Precision Journalism*.
3. "SRP [Savannah River Plant] link to diseases not valid," *Atlanta Journal-Constitution*, August 14, 1983.
4. U.S. Surgeon General Richard Carmona, quoted by the *Washington Post*, June 28, 2006, in "U.S. Details Dangers of Secondhand Smoking." Details of the second-hand risk are in the surgeon's general report on smoking that was released at that time.
5. Jay A. Winsten, "Science and the Media: The Boundaries of Truth," *Health Affairs* (Spring 1985): 5–23.

2

The Certainty of Uncertainty

The only trouble with a sure thing is the uncertainty.

Author unknown

There are known knowns. These are things we know that we know. There are known unknowns. That is to say, there are things that we now know we don't know. But there are also unknown unknowns. These are things we do not know we don't know.

Donald Rumsfeld

Scientists keep changing their minds.

Pediatricians' advice on how to put a baby down to sleep has changed over time. The tummy position was first to go, and then even the side position was vetoed. Now it's on-the-back only, based on the latest research about reducing the risk of Sudden Infant Death Syndrome (SIDS).[1]

Vioxx hit the market in 1999 as a major advance to treat the pain from arthritis and other causes. Later, it was tested to see if it also could help prevent colon polyps (and thus colon cancer). Instead, that study found a major heart risk in people who had taken the drug for a while. Much of the controversy over Vioxx is about whether the heart risk should have been seen and acted on earlier. Vioxx was pulled from the market and research continues to identify any possible risks from other pain-relief drugs.[2]

News & Numbers: A Writer's Guide to Statistics, Third Edition. Victor Cohn and Lewis Cope with Deborah Cohn Runkle.
© 2012 Victor Cohn and Lewis Cope. Published 2012 by Blackwell Publishing Ltd.

Many experts once thought that postmenopausal hormone treatments could help protect women's hearts. Then a National Institutes of Health study made big headlines by concluding that long-term use of this treatment increased heart, stroke, and breast cancer risks. But debate still simmers over specifics.[3]

In another seesaw, experts continue to tell us that coffee is good for us or bad for us.[4]

And poor Pluto! It had long reigned as our solar system's ninth planet. Then astronomers discovered similar far-out orbiting bodies, and there was talk of granting them planethood status. And some pointed out that Pluto's orbit was not like that of the eight other planets. So the International Astronomical Union took a vote and decided to demote Pluto to a secondary dwarf category – shrinking our roster of planets to eight.[5]

To some people, all this changing and questioning gives science a bad name. Actually, it's science working just as it's supposed to work.

The first thing that you should understand about science is that it is almost always uncertain. The scientific process allows science to move ahead without waiting for an elusive "proof positive." Patients can be offered a new treatment at the point at which there's a good probability that it works. And decisions to prohibit the use of a chemical in household products can be made when there's a pretty good probability that it's dangerous.

How can science afford to act on less than certainty? Because science is a continuing story – always retesting ideas. One scientific finding leads scientists to conduct more research, which may support and expand on the original finding. In medicine, this often allows more and more patients to benefit. And in cosmology this can lead to a better understanding of the origins of our universe.

But in other cases, the continuing research results in modified conclusions. Or less often, in entirely new conclusions.

Remember when a radical mastectomy was considered the only good way to treat breast cancer? When doctors thought that stress and a spicy diet were the main causes of ulcers – before research demonstrated that the chief culprit is bacteria? These and many other treatments and beliefs once seemed right, then were dropped after statistically rigorous comparisons with new ideas.

In considering the uncertainty inherent in science, we can say one thing with virtual certainty: Surprise discoveries will alter some of today's taken-for-granted thinking in medicine and other fields.

Now let's take a deeper look at some of research that shows how scientists change their minds with new evidence:

The dietary fat study – The federal Women's Health Initiative conducted the largest study ever undertaken to see whether a low-fat diet could reduce the risk of cancer or heart disease. It involved 49,000 women, ages 50 to 79, who were followed for eight years. In the end, there was no difference in heart or cancer risks between the participants assigned to the low-fat diet and those who weren't.

But wait! A closer look showed that women on the low-fat diet hadn't cut back their fat intake as much as hoped. And the diet was designed to lower *total* fat consumption, rather than targeting specific types of fat. That was considered good advice when the study was planned, but experts now emphasize cutting back on saturated and other specific fats to benefit the heart.

So the big study didn't totally settle anything – except maybe to confirm how hard it is to get people to cut back on fatty foods. It certainty didn't provide an endorsement for low-fat diets in general, as many thought it would. But a chorus of experts soon proclaimed continuing faith in the heart-health advice to cut back on specific types of fats. And more research has indicated that certain fats may be good for you – like the fat in certain fish and in dark chocolate! More research will try to sort everything out. Please stay tuned.[6]

The Scientific Method

Let's pause and take a step-by-step look at the scientific way:

A scientist seeking to explain or understand something – be it the behavior of an atom or the effect of the oil spilled in the Gulf – usually proposes a hypothesis, then seeks to test it by experiment or observation. If the evidence is strongly supportive, the hypothesis may then become a theory or at some point even a law, such as the law of gravity.

A theory may be so solid that it is generally accepted.

Example: The theory that cigarette smoking causes lung cancer, for which almost any reasonable person would say the case has been proved, for all practical purposes.

The phrase "for all practical purposes" is important, for scientists, being practical people, must often speak at two levels: the strictly scientific level and the level of ordinary reason that we require for daily guidance.

Example of the two levels: In 1985, a team of 16 forensic experts examined the bones that were supposedly those of the Nazi "Angel of Death," Dr. Josef Mengele. Dr. Lowell Levine, representing the U.S. Department of Justice, then said, "The skeleton is that of Josef Mengele within a reasonable scientific certainty," and Dr. Marcos Segre of the University of São Paulo, explained, "We deal with the law of probabilities. We are scientists and not magicians." Pushed by reporters' questions, several of the pathologists said they had "absolutely no doubt" of their findings.[7] Yet the most that any scientist can scientifically say – say with certainty in almost any such case – is: There is a very strong probability that such and such is true.

"When it comes to almost anything we say," reports Dr. Arnold Relman, former editor of the *New England Journal of Medicine*, "you, the reporter, must realize – and must help the public understand – that we are almost always dealing with an element of uncertainty. Most scientific information is of a probable nature, and we are only talking about probabilities, not certainty. What we are concluding is the best we can do, our best opinion at the moment, and things may be updated in the future."

Example: In the beginning, all cholesterol that coursed the bloodstream was considered an artery-clogging heart hazard. Then researchers discovered that there's not only bad cholesterol, but also some good cholesterol that helps keep the arteries clean. Exercise, among other things, can help pump up the level of HDL (good cholesterol).

Just as Americans were taking this message to heart, the what-to-eat part of the cholesterol message began to change, too.

The chief concern had long focused on eating too much saturated fat, which is the type typically found in meats. Then, research in the 1990s uncovered growing worries about the consumption of "trans fats," an unusual form of vegetable fat that's typically found in some snack foods and some types of fried foods.

By 2006, when trans fats were added to food labels, some experts were calling this the worst of all fats for the heart. Recent research has shown that trans fats can both *lower* the bloodstream's level of *good* cholesterol, and *raise* the level of *bad* cholesterol.

Of course, research continues on all aspects of heart attack prevention, with hopes of coming up with new and better advice. So please stay tuned.[8]

Nature is complex, and almost all methods of observation and experiment are imperfect. "There are flaws in all studies," says Harvard's Dr. Marvin Zelen.[9] There may be weaknesses, often unavoidable ones, in the way a study is designed or conducted. Observers are subject to human bias and error. Measurements fluctuate.

"Fundamentally," writes Dr. Thomas Vogt, "all scientific investigations require confirmation, and until it is forthcoming all results, no matter how sound they may seem, are preliminary."[10]

But when study after study reaches the same conclusion, confidence can grow. Scientists call this *replication* of the findings. We call it the way that science grows by building on itself.

Even when the test of time provides overwhelming evidence that a treatment really does help, there may be questions about just which patients should get the treatment. These questions are arising more as we enter an age of "personalized medicine," in which patients with particular genetic profiles or other biological markers (called "biomarkers") are found to be better candidates for a treatment than others with the same disease. And if an "improved" treatment comes along, is the new treatment really an improvement? *Comparitive effectiveness research*, another type of medical research, aims to test one therapy against another to try to answer that question.

The bottom line for journalists covering all types of research: Good reporters try to tell their readers and viewers the degree of uncertainty, whether it's about a medical research finding or the effects of global warming. And wise reporters often use words such as "may" and "evidence indicates," and seldom use words like "proof." A newspaper or TV report or blog that contains needed cautions and caveats is a more credible report than one that doesn't.

Focusing on Medicine

Medicine, in particular, is full of disagreement and controversy. The reasons are many:

There's the lack of funds to mount enough trials. There's the swift evolution and obsolescence of some medical techniques.

There's the fact that, with the best of intentions, medical data – histories, physical exams, interpretations of tests, descriptions of symptoms and diseases – are too often inexact and vary from physician to physician.

There are ethical obstacles to trying a new procedure when an old one is doing some good, or to experimenting on children, pregnant women, or the mentally ill.

There may not be enough patients at any one center to mount a meaningful trial, particularly for a rare disease. And if there's a multicenter trial, there are added complexities and expenses.

And some studies rule out patients with "co-morbidities" – that is, diseases the patients have in addition to the one being studied – which might make for a purer result, but are usually not a reflection of the real world, where people often have more than one medical condition.

Studies have found that many articles in prestigious medical journals have shaky statistics, and a lack of any explanation of such important matters as patients' complications and the number of patients lost to follow-up. The editors of leading medical journals have gotten together and established standards for reporting clinical trials, so they will be of greater use to clinicians and other scientists. And most journals now have statisticians on their review boards. Research papers presented at medical meetings, many of them widely reported by the media, raise more questions. Some are mere progress reports on incomplete studies. Some state tentative results that later collapse. Some are given to draw comment or criticism, or to get others interested in a provocative but still uncertain finding.[11]

The upshot, according to Dr. Gary Friedman at the Kaiser organization's Permanente Medical Group: "Much of health care is based on tenuous evidence and incomplete knowledge."[12]

In general, possible risks tend to be underestimated and possible benefits overestimated. And studies have found that research that is funded by a drug's manufacturer show positive results for that drug more often than when a competing manufacturer or nonprofit, such as the government, is funding the study.[13] Occasionally, unscrupulous investigators falsify their results. More often, they may wittingly or unwittingly play down data that contradict their theories, or they may search out statistical methods that give them the results they want. Before ascribing fraud, says Harvard's Dr. Frederick Mosteller, "keep in mind the old saying that most institutions have enough incompetence to explain almost any results."[14]

But don't despair. In medicine and other fields alike, the inherent uncertainties of science need not stand in the way of good sense. To live – to survive on this globe, to maintain our health, to set public policy, to govern ourselves – we almost always must act on the basis of incomplete or uncertain information. There is a way we can do so, as the next two chapters explain.

Notes

1. http://kidshealth.org/parent/general/sleep/sids.html
2. "Arthritis Drug Vioxx Being Pulled Off Market," Reuters news service, September 30, 2004, and other news reports.

3. Tara Parker-Pope, "In Study of Women's Health, Design Flaws Raise Questions," *Wall Street Journal,* February 28, 2006; Laura Neergaard, Associated Press dispatch on controversies over studies, February 27, 2006; other news reports.

4. http://www.health.harvard.edu/press_releases/coffee_health_risk

5. http://news.nationalgeographic.com/news/2006/08/060824-pluto-planet.html

6. Gina Kolata, "Low Fat Diet Does Not Cut Health Risks, Study Finds," *New York Times,* February 8, 2006, and other news reports; see also note 3.

7. From many news reports, including "Absolutely No Doubt," *Time,* July 1, 1985.

8. "Trans Fat Overview," American Heart Association fact sheet; "Trans Fats 101," University of Maryland Medical Center fact sheet; Marian Burros, "KFC Is Sued Over the Use of Trans Fats in its Cooking," *New York Times,* June 14, 2006.

9. Marvin Zelen talk at Council for the Advancement of Science Writing (CASW) seminar "New Horizons of Science," Cambridge, Mass., November 1982.

10. Vogt, *Making Health Decisions.*

11. From many sources, including John T. Bruer, "Methodological Rigor and Citation Frequency in Patient Compliance Literature," *American Journal of Public Health* 72, no. 10 (October 1982): 1119–24; "Despite Guidelines, Many Lung Cancer Trials Poorly Conducted," *Internal Medicine News* (January 1, 1984); Rebecca DerSimonian et al., "Reporting on Methods in Clinical Trials," *New England Journal of Medicine* 306, no. 22 (June 3, 1982): 1332–37; Kenneth S. Warren in *Coping,* ed. Warren.

12. Friedman, *Primer.*

13. R. E. Kelly et al., "Relationship Between Drug Company Funding and Outcomes of Clinical Psychiatric Research," *Psychological Medicine* 36 (2006): 1647–56.

14. Frederick Mosteller in *Coping,* ed. Warren.

3

Testing the Evidence

The great tragedy of Science (is) the slaying of a beautiful hypothesis by an ugly fact.

Thomas Henry Huxley

A father noticed that every time any of his 11 kids dropped a piece of bread on the floor, it landed with the buttered side up. "This utterly defies the laws of chance," the father exclaimed.

He just needed to ask one good question: Is there some other explanation for this buttered-side-up phenomenon? Close examination disclosed that his kids were buttering both sides of their bread.

Experts call this the failure to consider an alternate explanation. We call it the need for clear thinking.

Other examples that illustrate the need to think clearly before reaching conclusions:

- You may say that there's only a one-in-a-million chance that something will happen today. But remember, "an event with a one-in-a-million chance of happening to any American on any given day will, in fact," occur about 300 times each day in this nation of some 300 million Americans, pointed out John Allen Paulos, a mathematics professor at Temple University.[1]

News & Numbers: A Writer's Guide to Statistics, Third Edition. Victor Cohn and Lewis Cope with Deborah Cohn Runkle.
© 2012 Victor Cohn and Lewis Cope. Published 2012 by Blackwell Publishing Ltd.

Experts call this the *Law of Small Probabilities*. We call it the Law of Unusual Events.

- Someone might look at professional basketball players and conclude that this sport makes people grow tall. Or look at the damage wreaked on mobile home parks by tornadoes, then conclude that mobile home parks cause tornadoes.[2]

Experts call this falsely concluding that association proves causation. We just call it crazy thinking.

Laugh if you must. These three examples illustrate the need to follow some of the basic principles of good statistical analysis.

How to Search for the Truth

As journalists, we talk to researchers, politicians, advocates, self-proclaimed experts, real experts, true believers, and others, including an occasional fraud who tries to fool us. We listen to their claims in fields ranging from science to education, criminal justice, economics, and many other areas of our lives.

How can we journalists tell the facts, or the probable facts, from misleading and mistaken claims? We can borrow from science. We can try to judge all possible claims of fact by the same methods and rules of evidence that scientists use to derive some reasonable guidance in scores of unsettled issues. As a start, we can ask:

- **How do you know?**
- **Have the claims been subjected to any studies or experiments?** Or are you just citing some limited evidence that suggests that a real study should be conducted?
- **If studies have been done, were they acceptable ones, by general agreement?** Were they without any substantial bias?
- **Are your results fairly consistent with those from related studies, and with general knowledge in the field?**
- **Have the findings resulted in a consensus among other experts in the same field?** Do at least the majority of informed persons agree? Or should we withhold (or strongly condition) our judgment until there is more evidence?

- **Are the conclusions backed by believable statistical evidence?** And what is the degree of certainty or uncertainty? How sure can you be?
- **Is there reasonable theoretical plausibility to the findings?** In other words, do you have a good explanation for the findings?

Most importantly, much of statistics involves clear thinking rather than numbers. And much, at least much of the statistical principles that reporters can most readily apply, is good sense.

There are many definitions of statistics as a tool. A few useful ones: The science and art of gathering, analyzing, and interpreting data. A means of deciding whether an effect is real, rather than the result of chance. A way of extracting information from a mass of raw data.

Statistics can be manipulated by charlatans and self-deluders. And good people make some mistakes along with their successes. And qualified statisticians can differ on the best type of statistical analysis in any particular situation. Deciding on the truth of a matter can be difficult for the best statisticians, and sometimes no decision is possible. In some situations, there will inevitably be some uncertainty and in all situations uncertainty is always lurking.

In some fields, like engineering, for some things no numbers are needed. "Edison had it easy," says Dr. Robert Hooke, a statistician and author. "It doesn't take statistics to see that a light has come on."[3] While examples in medicine are rare, it didn't take statistics to tell physicians that the first antibiotics cured infections that until then had been highly fatal.

Overwhelmingly, however, the use of statistics, based on probability, is called the soundest method of decision-making. And the use of large numbers of cases, statistically analyzed, is called the only means for determining the unknown cause of many events.

Example: Birth control pills were tested on several hundred women, yet the pills had to be used for several years by millions before it became unequivocally clear that some women would develop heart attacks or strokes. The pills had to be used for some years more before it became clear that the greatest risk was to women who smoked and women over 35.

The best statisticians, along with practitioners on the firing line (e.g., physicians), often have trouble deciding when a study is adequate or meaningful. Most of us cannot become statisticians, but we can at least learn that there are studies and studies, and that the unadorned claim that "we conducted a study" or "we did an experiment" may not mean much. We can learn to ask better questions if we understand some basic facts about scientific studies. Here are four bedrock statistical concepts:

1. **Probability** (including the Law of Unusual Events)
2. **"Power" and numbers**
3. **Bias and "other explanations"**
4. **Variability**

We'll take them one by one.

Probability and Unexpected Events

Scientists cope with uncertainty by measuring probabilities. All experimental results and all events can be influenced by chance, and almost nothing is 100 percent certain in science and medicine and life. So probabilities sensibly describe what has happened and should happen in the future under similar conditions. Aristotle said that the probable "is what usually happens," but he might have added that the improbable happens more often than most of us realize.

Statistical significance

The accepted numerical expression of probability in evaluating scientific and medical studies is the P (or *probability*) value. The P value is one of the most important figures a reporter should look for. It is determined by a statistical formula that takes into account the numbers of people or events being compared (more is better) to answer the question: Could a difference or result this great or greater have occurred just by chance alone?

A low P value means a low probability that chance alone was at work. It means, for example, that there is a low probability that a medical treatment might have been declared beneficial when in truth it was not.

In a nutshell, the lower the P value, the more likely it is that a study's findings are "true" results and not due to chance alone.

The P value is expressed either as an exact number or as $<.05$, say, or $>.05$. This means "less than" or "greater than" a 5 percent probability that the observed result could have happened just by chance – or, to use a more elegant statistician's phrase, by *random variation.*

Here is how the *P* value is used to evaluate results:

- By convention, a *P* value of .05 or less, meaning there are only 5 or fewer chances in 100 that the result could have happened by chance, is most often regarded as low. This value is usually called *statistically significant* (though sometimes other values are used). The unadorned term "statistically significant" usually implies that *P* is .05 or less.
- A higher *P* value, one greater than .05, is usually seen as not statistically significant. The higher the value, the more likely it is that the result is due to chance.

In common language and ordinary logic, a low likelihood of chance alone calling the shots means "it's close to certain." A strong likelihood that chance could have ruled means "it almost certainly can't be."

Why the number .05 or less? Partly for standardization. People have agreed that this is a good cutoff point for most purposes.

And partly out of common sense. Harvard's Mosteller tells us that if you toss a coin repeatedly in a college class and after each toss ask the class if there is anything suspicious going on, "hands suddenly go up all over the room" after the fifth head or tail in a row. There happens to be only one chance in 16 – .0625, not far from .05, or 5 chances in 100 – that five heads or tails in a row will show up in five tosses. "So there is some empirical evidence that the rarity of events in the neighborhood of .05 begins to set people's teeth on edge."[4]

Another common way of reporting probability is to calculate a *confidence level,* as well as a *confidence interval* (or *confidence limits* or *range*). This is what happens when a political pollster reports that candidate X would now get 50 percent of the vote and thereby leads candidate Y by 3 percentage points, "with a 3-percentage-point margin of error plus or minus at the 95 percent confidence level." In other words, Mr. or Ms. Pollster is 95 percent confident that X's share of the vote would be someplace between 53 and 47 percent. In a close election, that margin of error could obviously turn a candidate who is trailing in the poll into the election-day victor.

The larger the number of subjects (patients or other participants) in a study, the greater is the chance of a high confidence level and a narrow, and therefore more reassuring, confidence interval.

False positives, negatives, cause and effect

No matter how reassuring they sound, *P* values and confidence statements cannot be taken as gospel, for .05 is not a guarantee, just a number. There are important reasons for this:

- **False positives** – All that *P* values measure is the *probability* that the experimental results could be the product of chance alone. In 20 experiments that report a positive finding at a *P* value of .05, on average one of these findings will be the result of chance alone. This is called a false positive. For example, a treatment may appear to be helping patients when it really isn't.

Dr. Marvin Zelen pointed to the many clinical (patient) trials of cancer treatment underway today. If the conventional value of .05 is adopted as the upper permissible limit for false positives, then every 100 studies with no actual benefit may, on average, produce 5 false-positive results, leading physicians down false paths.[5]

Many false positives are discovered by follow-up studies, but others may remain unrecognized. Relatively few studies are done that exactly repeat original studies; scientists aren't keen on spending their time to confirm someone else's work, and medical journals aren't keen on publishing them. But treatments are usually retested to try modifications and to expand uses, or sometimes to try to settle controversies.

- **False negatives** – An unimpressive *P* value may simply mean that there were too few subjects to detect a real effect. This results in false negatives – missing an effective treatment (or some other effect or result) when it really exists.

In statistical parlance, by the way, a false positive is a Type I error (finding a result when it's not there), and a false negative is a Type II error (not finding a result when it is there).

- **Questions about cause and effect** – Statistical significance alone does not mean that there is cause and effect. *Association* or *correlation* is only a clue of possible cause.

Remember the rooster who thought he made the sun rise?
Just because a virus is found in patients with disease X doesn't mean it's the cause; the disease may have weakened their immune systems in a

way that allowed the virus to gain a foothold. Just because people who work with a chemical develop a disease doesn't mean that the chemical is the cause; the culprit may be something else in their workplace, or something not in the workplace at all that the workers have in common, like pollutants in the neighborhood in which they live.

In all such cases, more evidence is needed to confirm cause and effect (there is more about this in Chapter 5, "Cause-and-effect?"). To statisticians, by the way, association simply means that there is at least a possible relationship between two things. A correlation is a measure of the association.

- **"Significant" versus important** – Highly "significant" *P* values can sometimes adorn unimportant differences in large samples. An impressive *P* value might also be explained by some other variable or variables – other conditions or associations – not taken into account.

Also, statistical significance does not necessarily mean biological, clinical, or practical significance. Inexperienced reporters sometimes see or hear the word "significant" and jump to that conclusion, even reporting that the scientists called their study "significant."

Example: A tiny difference between two large groups in mean (or average) hemoglobin concentration, or red blood count, may be statistically significant yet medically meaningless.[6] **If the group is large enough, even very small differences can become statistically significant.**

And eager scientists can consciously or unconsciously "manipulate" the *P* value by choosing to compare different end points in a study (say, the patients' condition on leaving the hospital rather than length of survival) or by choosing the way the *P* value is calculated or reported.

There are several mathematical paths to a *P* value, such as the *chi-square,* the *t* test, the paired *t* test, and others. All can be legitimate. But be warned. Dr. David Salsburg, at Pfizer, Inc., has written in the *American Statistician* of the unscrupulous practitioner who "engages in a ritual known as 'hunting for *P* values.'" Such a person finds ways to modify the original data to "produce a rich collection of small *P* values" even if those that result from simply comparing two treatments "never reach the magical .05."[7]

A researcher at a major medical center contributes: "If you look hard enough through your data, if you do enough subset analyses, if you go through 20 subsets, you can find one" – say, "the effect of chemotherapy on pre-menopausal women with two to five lymph nodes" – "with a *P* value less than .05. And people do this." On the other hand, we're learning that these differences among subsets can sometimes be medically important.

"Statistical tests provide a basis for probability statements," writes the University of Chicago's Dr. John Bailar, "only when the hypothesis is fully developed before the data are examined ... If even the briefest glance at a study's results moves the investigator to consider a hypothesis not formulated before the study was started, that glance destroys the probability value of the evidence at hand." (At the same time, Bailar adds, "review of data for unexpected clues ... can be an immensely fruitful source of ideas" for new hypotheses "that can be tested in the correct way." And occasionally "findings may be so striking that independent confirmation ... is superfluous.")[8]

Expect some unexpected events

The laws of probability also teach us to expect some unusual, even impossible-sounding, events.

We've all taken a trip to New York or London or someplace and bumped into someone from home. The chance of that? We don't know, but if you and a friend tossed for a drink every day after work, the chance that your friend would ever win 10 times in a row is 1 in 1,024. Yet your friend would probably do so sometime in a four- or five-year period.

While we call it the Law of Unusual Events, statisticians call it the *Law of Small Probabilities*. By whatever name, it tells us that a few people with apparently fatal illnesses will inexplicably recover. It tells us that there will be some amazing clusters of cases of cancer or birth defects that will have no common cause. And it tells us that we may once in a great while bump into a friend far from home.

In a large enough population, such coincidences are not unusual. They produce striking anecdotes and often striking news stories. In the medical world, they produce unreliable, though often cited, testimonial or anecdotal evidence. "The world is large," Thomas M. Vogt notes, "and one can find a large number of people to whom the most bizarre events have occurred. They all have personal explanations. The vast majority are wrong."[9]

"We [reporters] are overly susceptible to anecdotal evidence," Philip Meyer writes. "Anecdotes make good reading, and we are right to use them ... But we often forget to remind our readers – and ourselves – of the folly of generalizing from a few interesting cases ... The statistic is hard to remember. The success stories are not."[10]

The Power of Big Numbers

This gets us to a related statistical concept of *power*. Statistically, power means the probability of finding something if it's there. For example, given that there is a true effect – say, a difference between two medical treatments or an increase in cancer caused by exposure to a toxin in a group of workers – how likely are we to find it?

Sample size confers power. Statisticians say, "There is no probability until the sample size is there" ... "Large numbers confer power" ... "Large numbers at least make us sit up and take notice."[11]

All this concern about sample size can also be expressed as the *Law of Large Numbers*, which says that as the number of cases increases, the probable truth – positive or negative – of a conclusion or forecast increases. The *validity* (truth or accuracy) and *reliability* (reproducibility) of the statistics begin to converge on the truth.

We already learned this when we talked about probability. But statisticians think of power as a function of both sample size and the accuracy of measurement, because that too affects the probability of finding something. Doing that, we can see that if the number of treated patients is small in a medical study, a shift from success to failure in only a few patients could dramatically decrease the success rate.

Example: If six patients have been treated with a 50 percent success rate, the shift to the failure column of just one patient would cut the success rate to 33 percent. And the total number is so small in any case that the result has little reliability. The result *might* be valid or accurate, but it would not be generalizable; in other words, we just don't know – it would not have reliability until confirmed by careful studies in larger samples.

The larger the sample, assuming there have been no fatal biases or other flaws, the more confidence a statistician would have in the result.

One science reporter said that he has a quick, albeit far from definitive, screening test that he calls "my rule of two": He often looks at the key numbers, then adds or subtracts two from them. For example, someone says there are five cases of some form of cancer among workers in a company. Would it seem meaningful if there were three?

A statistician says, "This can help with small numbers but not large ones." Mosteller contributes "a little trick I use a lot on counts of any size." He explains, "Let's say some political unit has 10,000 crimes or deaths or accidents this year ... That means the number may vary by a minimum of 200 every year without even considering growth, the business cycle, or any other effect. This will supplement your reporter's approach." More about this later in this chapter.

False negatives – missing an effect where there is one – are particularly common when there are small numbers.

"There are some very well conducted studies with small numbers, even five patients, in which the results are so clear-cut that you don't have to worry about power," says Dr. Relman. "You still have to worry about applicability to a larger population, but you don't have to doubt that there was an effect. When results are negative, however, you have to ask, How large would the effect have to be to be discovered?"

Many scientific and medical studies are underpowered – that is, they include too few cases. This is especially true if the disease or medical condition being studied is relatively uncommon. "Whenever you see a negative result," another scientist says, "you should ask, What is the power? What was the chance of finding the result if there was one?" One study found that an astonishing 70 percent of 71 well-regarded clinical trials that reported no effect had too few patients to show a 25 percent difference in outcome. Half of the trials could not have detected a 50 percent difference. This means that medically significant findings may have been overlooked.[12]

A statistician scanned an article on colon cancer in a leading journal. "If you read the article carefully," he said, "you will see that if one treatment was better than the other – if it would increase median survival by 50 percent, from five to seven and a half years, say – they had only a 60 percent chance of finding it out. That's little better than tossing a coin!"

The weak power of that study would be expressed numerically as .6, or 60 percent. Scan an article's fine print or footnotes, and you will *sometimes* find such a *power statement*.

How large is a large enough sample? One statistician calculated that a trial has to have 50 patients before there is even a 30 percent chance of finding a 50 percent difference in results.

Sometimes large populations indeed are needed.[13]

Examples: If some kind of cancer usually strikes 3 people per 2,000, and you suspect that the rate is quadrupled in people exposed to substance X, you would have to study 4,000 people for the observed excess rate to have a 95 percent chance of reaching statistical significance. The likelihood that a 30-to-39-year-old woman will suffer a myocardial infarction, or heart attack, while taking an oral contraceptive is about 1 in 18,000 per year. To be 95 percent sure of observing at least one such event in a one-year trial, you would have to observe nearly 54,000 women.[14]

Even the lack of an effect – sometimes called a *zero numerator* – can be a trap. Say someone reports, "We have treated 14 leukemic boys for five years with no resulting testicular dysfunction" – that is, zero abnormalities in 14. The question remains: How many cases would they have had to treat to have any real chance of seeing an effect? The more unusual the adverse effect, the greater is the number of cases that would have to be studied. The probability of an effect may be small yet highly important to know about. These numbers show how hard it is to study rare or unusual diseases or other events.

All this means that you often must ask: What's your *denominator*? What's the size of your population?[15] A disease rate of 10 percent in 20 individuals may not mean much. A 10 percent rate in 200 persons would be more impressive. A rate is only a figure. Always try to get both the numerator and the denominator.

The most important rule of all about any numbers: Ask for them. When anyone makes an assertion that should include numbers and fails to give them – when anyone says that most people, or even X percent, do such and such – you should ask: What are your numbers? After all, some researchers reportedly announced a new treatment for a disease of chickens by saying, "33.3 percent were cured, 33.3 percent died, and the other one got away."

Bias and Alternate Explanations

One scientist once said that lefties are overrepresented among baseball's heavy hitters. He saw this as "a possible result of their hemispheric lateralization, the relative roles of the two sides of the brain." A critic who had seen more ball games said some simpler covariables could explain the difference. When they swing, left-handed hitters are already on the move toward first base. And most pitchers are right-handers who throw most often to right-handed hitters, so these pitchers might not be quite as sharp throwing to lefty batters.[16]

Scientist A was apparently guilty of *bias,* which in science means the introduction of spurious associations and error by failing to consider other factors that might influence the outcome. The other factors may be called covariables, covariates, intervening or contributing variables, confounding variables, or confounders. In simpler terms, this means "other explanations."

Statisticians call bias "the most serious and pervasive problem in the interpretation of data from clinical trials" … "the central issue of epidemiological research" ... "the most common cause of unreliable data." Able and conscientious scientists try to eliminate biases or account for them in some way. But not everybody who makes a scientific, medical, or environmental claim is that skilled. Or that honest. Or that all-powerful. Some biases are unavoidable because of the degree of difficulty of a lot of research studies, and the most insidious biases of all, says one statistician, are "those we don't know exist."

A statistician recalled: "I was once called about a person who had won first, second, and third prizes in a church lottery. I was asked to assess the probability that this could have happened. I found out that the winner had bought nearly all the tickets." The statistician had, of course, asked the key question for both scientist and reporters: Could the relationship described be explained by other factors?

But bias is a pervasive human failing, and its effects often are more difficult to pin down.

Bias – in ordinary terms

One candid scientist is said to have admitted, "I wouldn't have seen it if I hadn't believed it."

Enthusiastic investigators often tell us their findings are exciting, and enthusiasm can be a good trait for scientists. But the findings may be so exciting that the investigators paint the results in over-rosy hues, forgetting needed caveats.

Other powerful human drives – the race for academic promotion and prestige, financial connections, obtaining grants – can also create conscious or unconscious attitudes that feed bias.

Two examples of where bias in the everyday-life meaning of the term may creep in:

Potential conflict of interest – Dr. Thomas Chalmers, at Mount Sinai Medical Center in New York, contrasts two drug trials, each sponsored by a pharmaceutical firm. In the first, the head of the study committee and the main statisticians and analysts were the firm's employees, though not so identified in any credits. In the second, the contract specifically called for a study protocol designed by independent investigators, and monitored by an outside board less likely to be influenced by a desire for a favorable outcome.

In fact, studies have shown that medical studies funded by pharmaceutical firms are more likely to emphasize positive results for their drug than those funded with public or other noncommercial money or those funded by a competitor.[17] David Michaels reports a similar phenomenon in a variety of research areas, for instance, toxicity studies. He reports that the difference in outcomes cannot be accounted for by scientists "fiddling" with the results in industry-funded research, but rather the important variable was study design, asking the "right" question from the outset.[18]

By the way, conflicts of interest can result from factors other than commercial or financial incentives. Sometimes a researcher's deeply held ideological or other beliefs can affect how research is conducted and reported. Thomas Mills and Roger Clark note that whether scientists can be advocates for a policy position "without compromising their role as an impartial provider" of information is "hotly debated."[19] John Weins, at Colorado State University, says that one's values can "really affect the way you design a study."[20] And Thomas Lovejoy, a strong supporter of the scientist as advocate, nevertheless warns that scientists in this role must be careful to "protect our capacity for self-criticism" that is so essential for good research.[21] For example, in an article on home births, the author tells us that advocates for having babies at home report that the moms recover faster, are more likely to breast feed, and less likely to suffer from postpartum depression. Was a study even conducted? We're not told. And the observer/reporters are likely to be biased. So be just as careful in telling your readers about advocacy group support for a science report as you would commercial support.

"It is never possible to eliminate" potential conflicts of interest in biomedical research, Chalmers concludes, but they should be disclosed so that others can evaluate them.[22]

Finding what you expect to find, even if it's wrong – For years, technicians computing blood counts were guided by textbooks that told them two or more "properly" studied samples from the same blood should not vary beyond narrow "allowable" limits. Reported counts always stayed inside those limits. A Mayo Clinic statistician rechecked and found that at least two-thirds of the time the discrepancies exceeded the supposed limits. The technicians had been seeing what they had been told to expect, and discounting any differences as their own mistakes. Perhaps coincidentally, this also saved them from the additional labor of doing still more counting.

Workers, placebos, and samples

We add to our watch-out-for list:

The healthy-worker effect – Occupational studies often confront a seeming paradox: The workers exposed to some possible adverse effect turn out to be healthier than the general population. The confounder: the well-known *healthy-worker effect*. Workers tend to be healthier and live longer than the population in general. The simple reason: They normally have to be healthy to get their jobs in the first place, and then they must stay relatively healthy to keep their jobs. The healthy-worker effect can mislead you into thinking that a workplace is safer than it really is.

The placebo effect and related phenomena – Both the *biased observer* and the *biased subject* are common in medicine. A researcher who wants to see a positive treatment result may see one. Patients may report one out of eagerness to please the researcher and to have a better disease outcome. There is also the powerful *placebo effect*. Summarizing many studies, one scientist found that half the patients with headaches or seasickness – and a third of those with coughs, mood changes, anxiety, the common cold, and even the disabling chest pains of angina pectoris – reported relief from a "nothing pill."[23]

A placebo is not truly a nothing pill. The mere expectation of relief seems to trigger important effects within the body in some people. But in a careful study, the placebo should not do as well as a test medication. Otherwise the test medication is no better than a placebo.

Sampling bias – This can be a bugaboo of both political polls (see Chapter 11) and medical studies. Say you want to know what proportion of the populace has heart disease, so you stand on a corner and ask people as they pass. Your sample is biased, if only because it leaves out those too disabled to get around. Your problem, a statistician would say, is *selection*.[24]

Other examples: A doctor in a clinic or hospital with an unrepresentative patient population – healthier or sicker or richer or poorer than average – may report results that do not represent the population as a whole. Veterans Affairs (VA) hospitals, for example, treat relatively few women. Their conclusions may apply only to the disproportionate number of lower-income men who typically seek out the VA hospitals' free care.

A celebrated Mayo or Cleveland or Ochsner clinic sees both a disproportionate number of difficult cases and a disproportionate number of patients who are affluent and well enough to travel.

Hence the importance of multicenter studies discussed above.

Don't be led astray

Age and other key variables – Age, gender, occupation, nationality, race, income, socioeconomic status, health status, and powerful behaviors such as smoking are all possible confounding – and frequently ignored – variables.

Three examples, each making a different point:

- *Exonerating a suspect* – In the 1970s, foes of adding fluoride to city water pointed to crude cancer mortality rates in 2 groups of 10 U.S. cities. One group had added fluoride to water, the other had not, and from 1950 to 1970 the cancer mortality rate rose faster in the fluoridated cities. The federal National Cancer Institute pointed out that the two groups were not equal: The difference in cancer deaths was almost entirely explained by differences in age, race, and gender. The age-, race-, and gender-adjusted difference actually showed a small, unexplained lower mortality rate in the fluoridated cities.[25]
- *Occupation, race or some other factor?* – Some studies of workers in steel mills showed no overall increase in cancer, despite possible exposures to various carcinogens. But lumping all workers together can mask other important factors. It took a look at African American workers alone to find excess cancer. They commonly worked at the coke ovens, where carcinogens were emitted. Such findings in African Americans often may be falsely ascribed to race or genetics. The real, or at least the most important, contributing or ruling variables – to a statistician, the *independent variables* – may be occupation and the social and economic plights that put African Americans in vulnerable settings. The excess cancer is the *dependent variable*, the result.

"In a two-variable relationship," Dr. Gary Friedman explains, "one is usually considered the independent variable, which affects the other or dependent variable."[26]

- *Diseases with multiple causes* – We know that more people get colds in winter than at other times of the year. Weather is commonly seen as the underlying or independent variable that affects the incidence of the common cold, the dependent variable. Actually, of course, some people, like children in school who are constantly exposed to new viruses, are more vulnerable to colds than others. In the case of these children, there is often more than one independent variable.

Thus, some people think that an important underlying reason for the prevalence of colds in winter may be that children are congregated in school, giving colds to each other, thence to their families, thence to their families' coworkers, thence to the coworkers' families, and so on. But cold weather and home heating may still figure, perhaps by drying nasal passages and making them more vulnerable to viruses.

The search for *true variables* is obviously one of the main pursuits of the epidemiologist, or disease detective – or of any physician who wants to know what has affected a patient, or of anyone who seeks true causes. Like colds, many medical conditions, such as heart disease, cancer, and probably mental illness, often have multiple contributing factors.

Where many known, measurable factors are involved, statisticians can use mathematical techniques to account for all the variables and try to find which are the truly important predictors. The terms for this include multiple regression, multivariate analysis, and discriminant analysis, and factor, cluster, path, and two-stage least-squares analyses.

Also remember: Smoking has been an important confounder in studies of industrial contaminants, in which the smokers suffer a disproportionate number of ill effects.[27] Or workers in some industries or occupations are more likely to be smokers than the overall population. Additionally, smoking plus an industrial contaminant may act synergistically, such that the two together have a multiplying effect on disease susceptibility.

Dropouts and other missing data – An investigator may also introduce bias by *constraining*, or distorting, a sample – by failing to reveal *nonresponse rates* or by otherwise "throwing away data."

Example: A surgeon cites his success rate in those discharged from the hospital after an operation, but omits those who died during or just after the procedure.

Many people drop out of studies. Sometimes they just quit. Or they are dropped for various reasons: They could not be evaluated, they came down with some "irrelevant" disorders, they moved away, they died. In fact, many of those not counted may have had unfavorable outcomes had they stayed in the study. There are statistical methods that try to account for these "missing" subjects, but they may not always be used.

The presence of significant nonresponse can often be detected, when reading medical papers, by counting the number of patients treated versus the number of untreated or differently treated controls – patients with whom the treated patients are compared. If the number of controls is strikingly greater in a randomized clinical trial (though not necessarily in an epidemiological or environmental study), there may have been many dropouts. A well-conducted study should describe and account for them. A study that does not may report a favorable treatment result by ignoring the fate of the dropouts.

For two excellent examples of alternate explanations, see "Family Life" and "Religion" in Chapter 12.

Variability

Regression toward the mean is the tendency of all values in every field of science – physical, biological, social, and economic – to move toward the average. Tall fathers tend to have sons shorter than they are, and short fathers, taller sons. The students who get the highest grades on an exam tend to get somewhat lower ones the next time. The regression effect is common to all repeated measurements.

Regression is part of an even more basic phenomenon: *variation*, or *variability*. Virtually everything that is measured varies from measurement to measurement. When repeated, every experiment has at least slightly different results.

Examples: Take a patient's blood pressure, pulse rate, or blood count several times in a row, and the readings will be somewhat different. The important reasons? In part, fluctuating physiology, but also the limits of measurement accuracy, and observer variation. Examining the same patient, no two doctors will report exactly the same results, and the results may be very different.

If six doctors examine a patient with a faint heart murmur, only one or two may have the skill or keen hearing to detect it. Experimental results so typically differ from one time to the next that scientific and medical fakers – a Boston cancer researcher, for example – have been detected by the unusual regularity of their reported results. Their numbers agree too well and the same results appear time after time, with not enough variation from patient to patient.

Biological variation is the most important cause of variation in physiology and medicine. Different patients, and the same patients, react differently to the same treatment. (Scientists are studying this phenomenon to try to determine what accounts for the different treatment responses.) Disease rates differ in different parts of the country and among different populations, and – alas, nothing is simple – there is natural variation within the same population.

Every population, after all, is a collection of individuals, each with many characteristics. Each characteristic, or *variable*, such as height, has a *distribution* of values from person to person, and – if we would know something about the whole population – we must have some handy summaries of the distribution. We can't get much out of a list of 10,000 measurements, so we need single values that summarize many measurements.

Average and related numbers – The *mean, median,* and *mode* can give us some idea of the look of the whole and its many measurable properties, or *parameters.*

When most of us speak of an average, we mean simply the *mean* or *arithmetic average,* the sum of all the values divided by the number of values. The mean is no mean tool; it is a good way to get a typical number, but it has limitations, especially when there are some extreme values.

Example: There is said to be a memorial in a Siberian town to a fictitious Count Smerdlovski, the world's champion at Russian roulette. On the average he won, but his actual record was 73 and 1.[28]

If you look at the arithmetic average of salaries in Company X, you will not know that a third of the personnel are working for the minimum wage, while a few make $100,000 or more a year. You may learn more here from the *median* – which is the midpoint in a list of figures. You also can think of the median as the middle value. In Company X, the median salary is $30,000 a year; half the employees earn that much or less, and the other half earn that much or more.

The median can be of value when a group has a few members with extreme values, like the 400-pounder at an obesity clinic whose other patients weigh from 180 to 200 pounds. If he leaves, the patients' mean weight might drop by 10 pounds, but the median might drop just 1 pound.[29]

The most frequently occurring number or value in a distribution is called the *mode.* When the median and the mode are about the same – or even more when mean, median, and mode are roughly equal – you can feel comfortable about knowing the typical value. When plotted on a graph, this is a *bell curve.*

With many of the things that scientists, economists, or others measure and then plot on a graph – test scores are just examples – we typically tend to see a familiar, bell-shaped *normal distribution,* high in the middle and low at each end, or *tail.* This bell curve is also called a *Gaussian curve,* named after the 19th-century German mathematician Karl Friedrich Gauss.

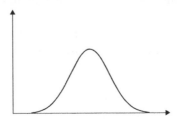

The normal distribution.

Range and distribution – You still need to know something about the exceptions, in short, the *dispersion* (or spread or scatter) of the entire distribution. One measure of spread is the *range*. It tells you the lowest and highest values. It might inform you, for example, that the annual salaries in a company range from $10,000 to $250,000.

You can also divide your values into 100 *percentiles*, so you can say someone or something falls into the 10th or 71st percentile, or into *quartiles* (fourths) or *quintiles* (fifths). One useful measure is the *interquartile range*, the interval between the 75th and 25th percentiles – this is the distribution in the middle, which avoids the extreme values at each end. Or you can divide a distribution into subgroups – those with incomes from $10,000 to $20,000, for example, or ages 20 to 29, 30 to 39, and so on.

Standard deviation – A widely used number, the *standard deviation*, can reveal a great deal. No matter how it sounds, it is not the average distance from the mean, but a more complex figure. Unlike the range, this handy figure takes full account of every value to tell how spread out things are – how dispersed the measurements.

Here's what one statistician calls a truly remarkable generalization: In most sets of measurement "and without regard to what is being measured," only 1 measurement in 3 will deviate from the average by more than 1 standard deviation, only 1 in 20 by more than 2 standard deviations, and only 1 in 100 by more than 2.57 standard deviations.

"Once you know the standard deviation in a normal, bell-shaped distribution," according to the University of Minnesota's Thomas Louis, "you can draw the whole picture of the data. You can visualize the shape of the curve without even drawing the picture, since the larger the variation of the numbers, the larger the standard deviation and the more spread out the curve – and vice versa."

Example: If the average score of all students who take the SAT college entrance test is relatively low and the spread – the standard deviation – is relatively large, this creates a very long-tailed, low-humped curve of test scores, ranging, say, from around 300 to 2,400. But if the average score of a group of brighter students entering an elite college is high, the standard deviation of the scores will be less and the curve will be high-humped and short-tailed, going from maybe 900 to 1,500. More about statistics and SAT scores in a later chapter.

"If I just told you the means of two such distributions, you might say they were the same," another scientist says. "But if I reported the means and the standard deviations, you'd know they were different, with a lot more variations in one."

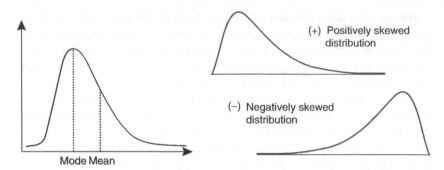

A skewed distribution.   Positively and negatively skewed distributions.

Distributions are not always normal, however. Some distributions are *skewed*, and are characterized by having most of the measurements (the mode) at one end of the curve, with an extended tail, of varying lengths, at the other end. Unlike a bell curve or normal distribution, the mode and mean of a skewed distribution are not the same. Skewed distributions can be *positively* or *negatively* skewed. For example, you might get a positively skewed curve when plotting survival times for certain severe cancers. That is, most of the patients die relatively soon after diagnosis, with fewer living for more extended times. Conversely, a negatively skewed curve could result if you plot SAT scores for students entering a highly selective university. Most of the scores are clustered near the top, with a tail of lower scores extending to the left of the curve.

Putting a human face on variability

From a human standpoint, variation tells us that it takes more than averages to describe individuals. Biologist Stephen Jay Gould learned in 1982 that he had a serious form of cancer. The literature told him the median survival was only eight months after discovery. Three years later, he wrote in *Discover*, "All evolutionary biologists know that means and medians are the abstractions," while variation is "the reality," meaning "half the people will live longer" than eight months.

Because he was young, because his disease had been diagnosed early, and because he would receive the best possible treatment, he decided he had a good chance of being at the far end of the curve. He calculated that the curve must be skewed well to the right, as the left half of the distribution had to be "scrunched up between zero and eight months, but the upper right half [could] extend out for years."

34

He concluded, "I saw no reason why I shouldn't be in that ... tail ... I would have time to think, to plan and to fight." Also, because he was being placed on an experimental new treatment, he might, if fortune smiled, "be in the first cohort of a new distribution with ... a right tail extending to death by natural causes at advanced old age."[30]

In 1999 – 17 years after the discovery of his cancer! – Gould became president of the American Association for the Advancement of Science, the world's largest membership organization representing all scientific disciplines. Gould lived for 20 years after his original diagnosis of cancer, dying in 2002 at age 60, of an apparently unrelated malignancy.

Statistics cannot tell us whether fortune will smile, only that such reasoning is sound.

Notes

1. John Allen Paulos, mathematics professor at Temple University, op-ed page article, *New York Times*, November 2, 1999.
2. Robert Young, Fox Chase Cancer Center, Philadelphia, personal communication.
3. Robert Hooke, *How to Tell the Liars From the Statisticians* (New York: Marcel Dekker, 1983).
4. Mosteller talk at the Council for the Advancement of Science Writing seminar "New Horizons of Science."
5. Zelen, "Innovations in the Design of Clinical Trials in Breast Cancer," in *Breast Cancer Research and Treatment*, no. 3 (1983), Proceedings of the Fifth Annual San Antonio Breast Cancer Symposium.
6. Friedman, *Primer*.
7. David S. Salsburg, "The Religion of Statistics as Practiced in Medical Journals," *American Statistician* 39, no. 3 (August 1985): 220–22.
8. John Bailar, "Science, Statistics and Deception," *Annals of Internal Medicine* 104, no. 2 (February 1986): 259–60.
9. Vogt, *Making Health Decisions*.
10. Meyer, *Precision Journalism*.
11. There is another unrelated use of the word "power." Scientists commonly speak of increasing or raising some quantity *by a power of* 2, or 3, or 100, or whatever. "Power" here means the product you get when you multiply a number by itself one or more times. Thus, in 2×2, number 2 has been raised to the second power. In $2 \times 2 \times 2$, number 2 has been raised to the third power to get a total of 8. When you think about 200 to the 100th power, you see the need for the shorthand.

12. J. A. Freiman, cited by Mosteller in *Coping*, ed. Warren.
13. Alvin R. Feinstein, "Epidemiology: Challenges and Controversies," in *1983 Encyclopedia Britannica Medical and Health Annual* (Chicago: Encyclopedia Britannica, 1983).
14. David L. Sackett in *Clinical Trials*, ed. Shapiro and Louis.
15. To a statistician, a population doesn't necessarily mean a group of people. Statistically, a population is any group or collection of pertinent units – units with one or more pertinent characteristics in common. They may be people, events, objects, records, test scores, or physiological values (such as blood pressure readings). Statisticians also use the term universe for a whole group of people or units under study.
16. David Hemenway, quoted in a Harvard School of Public Health staff newsletter, November 1983.
17. See Chapter 2, note 13.
18. David Michaels, "It's Not the Answers That Are Biased, It's the Questions," *Washington Post*, July 15, 2008.
19. Thomas Mills and Roger Clark, "Roles of Research Scientists in Natural Resource Decision Making," *Forest Ecology and Management* 153 (2001): 189–98.
20. Jocelyn Kaiser, "Ecologists on a Mission to Save the World," *Science* 287 (2000): 1188.
21. Thomas Lovejoy, "The Obligations of a Biologist," *Conservation Biology* 3 (1989): 329–30.
22. Thomas Chalmers in *Clinical Trials*, ed. Shapiro and Louis.
23. Henry K. Beecher, *Measurement of Subjective Responses: Quantitative Effects of Drugs* (New York: Oxford University Press, 1959).
24. Vogt, *Making Health Decisions*.
25. Hooke, *How to Tell the Liars*.
26. Friedman, *Primer*.
27. Department of Health, Education and Welfare, *The Health Consequences of Smoking: A Report of the Surgeon General*, 1980.
28. James Trefil, "Odds are Against Your Beating that Law of Averages," *Smithsonian* (September 1984): 66–75.
29. Friedman, *Primer*.
30. Stephen Jay Gould, "The Median Isn't the Message," *Discover* (June 1985): 40–42.

4

What Makes a Good Study?

If you want to inspire confidence, give plenty of statistics. It does not matter that they should be accurate, or even intelligible, as long as there is enough of them.

Lewis Carroll

The big problems with statistics, say its best practitioners, have little to do with computations and formulas. They have to do with judgment – how to design a study, how to conduct it, then how to analyze and interpret the results. Journalists reporting on statistics have many chances to do harm by shaky reporting, and so are also called on to make sophisticated judgments. How, then, can we tell which studies seem credible, which we should report?

Different problems require different methods, different numbers. One of the most basic questions in science is: Is the study designed in a way that will allow the researchers to answer the questions that they want answered?

We'll start with two case histories. The first comes from a clinical study of a drug, the second from an epidemiological study of a disease outbreak. The first led to unfounded hopes. The second is a short detective story with a surprise ending.

Case study 1: Physicians at a prestigious New England university used catheters to slowly infuse a theoretically promising drug into the

News & Numbers: A Writer's Guide to Statistics, Third Edition. Victor Cohn and Lewis Cope with Deborah Cohn Runkle.
© 2012 Victor Cohn and Lewis Cope. Published 2012 by Blackwell Publishing Ltd.

skulls of four Alzheimer's patients. According to the patients' families, three of the patients improved and the fourth at least held his own.

The university held a news conference, with one of the patients brought forth for an on-camera testimonial. The researcher used cautious words, but some newspaper headlines didn't. The story flew far and wide. The medical center got 2,600 phone calls, mainly from families of Alzheimer's patients who were desperate for any glimmer of hope.

There are two big reasons to question this study. A study of just four patients usually means little. A study whose effectiveness is judged by desperate family members is highly suspect. Not surprisingly, further study found that the drug didn't work.

Of course, many good studies are responsible for the many, many drugs and other new treatments that have revolutionized medicine and saved countless lives.

But in the four-patient Alzheimer's study, Harvard's Dr. Jay Winsten concluded, "The visual impact of [one] patient's on-camera testimonials all but guaranteed that TV coverage would oversell the research, despite any qualifying language."[1]

That said, sometimes even very small sample sizes can be highly suggestive, especially when the outcome being measured is objective, not subjective as in the Alzheimer's study. For example, in one study, two animals were infected with HIV and then infused with an antibody that blocks an important receptor. These animals didn't become infected, although the single animal that only got the virus and not the antibody did become infected. Whether an animal is infected or not is an objective laboratory finding, so this study, small as it is, gives us a strong clue that something meaningful may be going on.[2]

Case study 2: Minnesota Department of Health epidemiologists investigated a large outbreak of hepatitis A at a country club outing in 1978. They interviewed many of the more than 100 people who had become ill after eating at the club and, for comparison purposes, some who ate there but hadn't become ill.

This case-control study discovered a strong statistical association between eating hot dogs and becoming ill. But wait a minute! The cooking of the hot dog meat should have killed the hepatitis virus.

The problem turned out *not* to be the hot dogs. But the study had put the epidemiologists on the right track. Lab tests found the virus in the relish that people put on their hot dogs.

Further study discovered that a food worker who was handling the relish carried the hepatitis A virus. He found other work until he no longer was infectious. The cases of hepatitis stopped.[3] More about the great benefits, as well as limits, of case-control studies in a moment.

Epidemiology has its problems and controversies along with its many, many successes. The cause or causes of Gulf War Syndrome still stir debate, for example. And while epidemiologists led the way in showing preventive strategies for AIDS, some critics charged that progress was slow at the start of that epidemic.

Now epidemiologists are on guard for what *might* become a pandemic of the "bird flu" strain of influenza, or the "swine flu" that originated in Mexico. We emphasize "might," and will focus on this threat later in this chapter.

Together, clinical trials (also called clinical studies or patient trials) and epidemiological studies cover virtually the entire spectrum of health care.

Clinical trials evaluate drugs and other treatments, vaccines, and diagnostic procedures by testing them in humans, to see what will work and what won't.

Epidemiological studies probe the patterns and causes of all sorts of diseases and other health risks. These studies seek the answers that can prevent or limit future cases, so that we can live longer, healthier lives.

Before getting to the details of clinical and epidemiological studies, let's step back for a broader view and some history.

Experiments Versus Seductive Anecdotes

Scientific evidence can be weighed according to what's been called a hierarchy of evidence. Some kinds of studies carry more weight than others.

Science and medicine started with anecdotes, unreliable as far as generalization is concerned, yet provocative. Anecdotes matured into systematic observation. Simple eyeballing has developed into data collection and the recording of case histories. These are indispensable methods, yet still only one part of science. Case histories may not be typical, or they may reflect the beholder. Medicine continues to be plagued by big authorities who insist, "I know what I see."

There can still be useful, even inspired, observation and analysis of *natural experiments*. Excess fluoride in some waters hardened teeth, and this observation provided the first clue that fluoridation of drinking water might prevent tooth decay.

In 1585 or so, Galileo dropped weights from a tower and helped invent the *scientific experiment*. This means a study in which the experimenter controls the conditions and records the effect. Experiments on objects, animals, germs, and people matured into the modern experimental study, in which the experimenter changes only one thing, or some precisely planned number of things, to see how this affects the outcome.

It's a step-by-step process that, when done right, is done with care. Take a new potential treatment. First, the scientist has an idea, often based on previous research, about what might be *biologically plausible* and, thus, worth testing. Typically, the actual research starts in laboratory dishes or other lab apparatus, where it's relatively easy (and safe) to make changes. Then the research, if promising, may progress to animal trials. Yes, we must question whether specific lab and animal findings apply to humans. But very often animals provide a good substitute or "model" for human diseases, and it's too risky – and illegal – to test a drug on a human before sufficient animal studies have been conducted. But these questions can only be answered if the research progresses to, and then passes, the next step: clinical trials – that is, trials in people.

(Even if the clinical trials don't work out, that doesn't mean that the preceding laboratory and animal studies were in vain. They provide a growing store of knowledge that may lead to future research, with the potential for new treatment approaches or for new prevention strategies. In addition, research that may not appear to have any human applications may turn out otherwise. Studies of retrovirus in animals were extremely helpful when they demonstrated that HIV, the virus that causes AIDS, is a retrovirus. As we noted in Chapter 2, science is always building on itself. And this can happen in unpredictable ways.)

At each step along the way, all conscientious studies have one guiding principle: Each has a careful *design*. That is, it has the method or plan of attack that includes the right kind and number of patients or animals or in vitro studies, studies that occur in a laboratory vessel, not a living being. And it also tries to eliminate bias. Different kinds of studies require different methods. So one of the basic questions for a researcher is: Can this kind of experiment, this design, yield the answers I seek?

Clinical Researchers at Work

Experimental medicine's "gold standard" is the controlled, randomized clinical trial.[4] At its best, the investigator tests a treatment or drug or some other intervention by randomly selecting at least two comparable groups of people, the *experimental group* that is tested or treated and a *control group* that is observed for comparison.

A few of many possible examples: Randomized clinical trials proved that new drugs could cut the heart attack death rate, that treating hypertension could prevent strokes, and that polio, measles, and hepatitis vaccines worked. No doctor, observing a limited number of patients, could have shown these things.

Good clinical trials are expensive and difficult. It has been estimated that of 100 scheduled trials, 60 are abandoned, not implemented, or not completed. This may be for lack of funds, difficulty in recruiting or keeping patients, toxicity caused by the experimental drug or other problems, or, sometimes, rapid evidence of a difference in positive effect (making continued denial of effective treatment to patients in a control group unethical). Another 20 trials produce no noteworthy results, and just 20 have results worth publishing.

In fact, methodical research demonstrated that up to 37 percent of clinical trials that were reported in abstracts never were published as a full journal article.[5] Some authors thus concluded that health care and policy decisions had to rely on an incomplete and likely biased subset of clinical interventions.[6] To avoid this "selective" publication, the U.S. government set up a repository for the reporting of *all* clinical trials. How well is this working? There's some debate, but one author reports that fewer than half of published trials are registered and that studies sponsored by industry, as opposed to the NIH, have the worst publication record.[7]

Types of studies – Clinical studies can be classified by how a treatment is evaluated:

- Among the most reliable are *parallel studies* comparing similar groups given different treatments, or a treatment versus no treatment. But such studies are not always possible.
- In *crossover studies*, the same patients get two or more treatments in succession and act as their own controls. Similarly, *self-controlled studies* evaluate an experimental treatment by controlled observations during periods of no treatment or of some standard treatment.

There are potential pitfalls here. Treatment A might affect the outcome of treatment B, despite the usual use of a washout period between study periods. (This is why studies often randomly assign patients, so that some take treatment A first and others start with treatment B.) Patients become acclimated: They may become more tolerant of pain or side effects or, now more health-conscious, may change their ways.

The patients in a control group don't always behave in parallel studies either. In one large-scale trial of methods to lower blood cholesterol and the risk of heart disease, many controls adopted some of the same methods – quitting cigarette smoking, eating fewer fats – and reduced their risk too.

- Investigators often use *historical controls*, which means comparison with old records. Historically, the cure rate has been 30 percent, say, and the new therapy cures 60 percent. Or researchers use other *external controls* (such as comparison with other studies). These controls are often misleading. The groups compared aren't always comparable. The treatments may have been given by different methods. Laboratories may differ in their method of analyzing tissue samples. But this approach is still at times useful.

Historical controls often are used for nonclinical studies too. *Examples*: Researchers want to see the effect of an increase in cigarette taxes on smokers; the researchers compare smoking rates and cigarette sales before and after the tax increase. Researchers want to look at the effect of lowering the highway speed limit; they compare before-and-after accident rates. But always ask: Were there any other changes that might have affected the smoking rates, the accident rate, or whatever is being studied?

Judging clinical studies

All studies, including the best, have potential pitfalls. Here's a look at what makes clinical studies – and in some cases other types of studies too – as good as they can be:

1. **Adequate controls are needed** if you want to put the results in the bank.
2. **The number of patients must be large enough,** whether 10 or 10,000, to get trustworthy results, and representative enough so that the findings will apply to a larger population. Because people vary so widely in their reactions, and a few patients can fool you, fair-sized groups of patients are usually needed. Picking patients for a medical study is similar to picking citizens to be questioned in a political poll. In both, a sample is studied and inferences – the results in patients in general, the outcome of an election – are made for a larger population.

To get a large enough sample, medical researchers can conduct *multicenter trials*. Such trials are appealing because they can include hundreds of patients, but expensive and tricky because one must try to maintain similar selection and quality control at 10 institutions, maybe even 100 institutions. This approach also helps guard against institutional or regional bias. Successful multicenter trials established the value of controlling hypertension to prevent strokes and demonstrated the strong probability that less extensive surgery, the so-called *lumpectomy*, is as effective as more drastic surgery for many breast cancer patients.

3. **The patients should be randomized,** that is, divided by some random method into experimental and control groups. Randomization can easily be violated. A doctor assigning patients to treatment A or B may, seeing a particular type of patient, say or think, "This patient will be better on B."

   If treatment B has been established as better than A, there should be no random study in the first place and certainly no study of that doctor's patient. When randomization is violated, "the trial's guarantee of lack of bias goes down the drain," says one critique. As a result, patients who consent to randomization are often assigned to study groups according to a list of computer-generated random numbers.

4. **"Blinding" can add much confidence to a study.** To combat bias in investigators or patients, studies should be blinded. To the extent feasible, they can be single-, double-, or, best of all, triple-blinded – so that neither the doctors nor the nurses administering a treatment, nor the patients, nor those who assess the results know whether today's pill is treatment A, treatment B, or an inactive placebo. Otherwise, a doctor or patient who yearns for a good result may see or feel one when the "right" drug is given. There is a tale of an overzealous receptionist who, knowing which patients were getting the real drug and not the placebo, was so encouraging to these patients that they began saying they felt good willy-nilly.[8]

   Barring observant receptionists, the use of a placebo – from the Latin "I shall please" – may help maintain "blindness." Placebos actually give some relief in a third of all patients, on the average, in various conditions. The effect is usually temporary, however, and a truly effective drug ought to work substantially better than the placebo.

   Blinding is often impossible or unwise. Some treatments don't lend themselves to it, particularly many types of surgery. And some drugs quickly reveal themselves by various "side" effects. But an unblinded test is a weaker test.

5. **The research findings need to be stratified,** to test them and to learn the most from them. That is, for analysis they are separated into groups by age, gender, socioeconomic status, and so on. This can combat the influence of confounding variables and can yield answers applicable to various populations. Failure to stratify can hide true associations in various types of studies. And today, at the beginning of the era of *personalized medicine,* patients may be stratified based on genetic or other molecular differences, to try to tease out why drugs often work on most patients, but not all of them.

    An example from a clinical study: A study of open-heart surgery patients may separate out those who had to wait for their surgery. Some patients die waiting; those left are relatively stronger patients who do better, on average, than those treated immediately after diagnosis.

    An example from personalized medicine: 20 to 30 percent of breast cancer tumors "overexpress" the HER2 gene, causing cancer cells to multiply at a faster rate than others. But the good news is that these women can be treated with a drug called Herceptin, while the drug will be ineffective for the other 70 to 80 percent.[9]

    An example from epidemiology: The role of high-absorbency tampons in toxic shock syndrome was clarified only when the cases were broken down by the precise types of tampon used. More about that in a moment.

    An example from economics: Even in times of high employment, breakdowns by age and race might show problem pockets of joblessness.

    Large studies are generally necessary for stratification. When researchers subdivide their findings, the numbers in each subgroup get smaller. If the subgroups are too small, power is lost – a finding may be missed.

6. **A good study is reported fairly and candidly** by the research team. Dr. John Bailar warns of practices that sometimes have much value but at other times are "inappropriate and improper and, to the extent that they are deceptive, unethical." Among them: The selective reporting of findings, leaving out some that might not fit the conclusion. The reporting of a single study in multiple fragments, when the whole might not sound so good. And the failure to report the low power of some studies, their inability to detect a result even if one existed.[10]

Alternative Medicine

Alternative (sometimes called complementary) medicine can involve herbal medications, a variety of stress-reduction techniques, acupuncture, and various other unconventional approaches. Some alternative approaches have been shown to help. More and more studies are being done to assess which others may help and which may not. Some adherents of alternative medicine claim that it should not be judged by traditional models. What standards should we use to judge these approaches?

Our belief: Alternative medicine and conventional medicine should be judged by the same standards, based on the results of rigorous clinical studies with sound numbers. Both affect our bodies and our pocketbooks, so we deserve no less.

Epidemiologists at Work

In earlier times, epidemiology was concerned wholly with epidemics like smallpox, typhoid, and other infections. In 1740, Percival Pott scored a famous epidemiological success by observing the high rate of scrotum cancer in London's chimney sweeps. He correctly blamed it on their exposure to soot-burned organic material, much like a smoked cigarette. A century later, John Snow, plotting London cholera cases on a map and noting a cluster around one source of drinking water, removed the handle from the now famous Broad Street pump and helped end a deadly epidemic.

In today's world of drug abuse and road rage, epidemics are no longer limited to diseases. The mandate of disease detectives – formally called epidemiologists – has widened to meet the new challenges.

Today, "Epidemiology cuts across all aspects of health and behavior, it involves all aspects of public health," said Dr. Michael Osterholm, former state epidemiologist for Minnesota, and now director of the Center for Infectious Disease Research and Policy at the University of Minnesota.

Today's epidemiologists still track down infectious diseases. They have found the causes of new scourges, such as toxic shock syndrome, Legionnaires' disease, and AIDS and of old scourges like salmonella. As they probe outbreaks of many old as well as some new illnesses, they promote prevention when the cause is known, and seek the cause when it is not yet known.

Today's epidemiologists also study noninfectious diseases, which have become the biggest killers in our modern world. Epidemiologists successfully indicted smoking as a cause of lung cancer and heart disease. They identified the association of fats and cholesterol with clogging of the heart's arteries, changing the way that some Americans eat. And they pointed the way to the nation's exercise boom as a means of improving health.

They also provide the human-toll figures and other evidence that stir political debates over issues ranging from gun control to buckling-up in your car. They study everything from environmental problems to the effects of stress, from child and maternal health to the problems of aging.

In all these many ways considered together, epidemiologists may affect how we live our lives more than any other scientists.

Just as with clinical studies, epidemiological studies follow the basic rules of scientific and statistical analysis described in earlier chapters. And just as with clinical studies, epidemiological studies can take different forms to tackle different questions.

All forms of epidemiological studies have value, and all have limits. All look for telltale patterns and other evidence that can bring the knowledge needed to control health-related problems. All seek preventive approaches or other strategies for better health.

Types of studies

Epidemiology, like all science, started with *observational studies*, and these remain important. These studies, without comparison groups, are uncertain when it comes to determining cause and effect. Yet observation is how we first learned of the unfortunate effects of toxic rain, Agent Orange, cigarette smoking, and many sometimes helpful, sometimes harmful medications.

Some observational studies are simply *descriptive* – describing the incidence, prevalence, and mortality rates of various diseases, for example. Other, *analytic* studies seek to analyze or explain: The Seven-Country Study, for example, helped associate high meat and dairy fat and cholesterol consumption with excess risk of coronary heart disease.

Ecological studies look for links between environmental conditions and illness.

Human migrations such as the Japanese who came to the United States, ate more fat, and developed more disease are *natural experiments*.

Many epidemiological surveys rely on *samples* to represent the whole. These include government surveys of health and nutritional habits, of driving patterns, and of drug abuse. Samples and surveys often use questionnaires to get information. But questionnaires are no better than the quality of the answers.

Example: One survey compared patients' reporting of their current chronic illnesses with those their doctors recorded. The patients failed to mention almost half of the conditions that the doctors detected over the course of a year.

Whether it comes to illness, diets, or drinking, people tend to put themselves in the best possible light. A survey may stand or fall on the use of sophisticated ways to get accurate information. (See Chapter 11 on polling techniques.)

Epidemiologists' studies may also be classified in other ways:

- A *prevalence study* is a wide-angle snapshot of a population. It's a look at the rate of disease X or health-related problem Z, and its possible effects by age, gender, or other variables. This also may be called a current or cross-sectional study.
- A *case-control study* examines cases, along with a control group, for an intense, close-up analysis of a disease's relationship to other factors. The case-control study is a great way to assemble clues, to focus the investigation. But more research often must follow to nail down the culprit. A good example is the hot dogs and relish case at the beginning of this chapter.

Other examples: The nation hears of cases of toxic shock syndrome, mainly in young women. Epidemiologists at the federal Centers for Disease Control and Prevention launch a field investigation to find a series of patients, or cases. The epidemiologists confirm the diagnosis, then interview the patients and their families and other contacts to assemble careful case histories that cover, hopefully, all possible causes or associations. This group is then compared with a randomly selected matched comparison (control) group of healthy young women of like age and other characteristics. The women who developed toxic shock were much more likely to have used tampons. But it took more study, by Osterholm and others, to show that the real risk was in high-absorbency tampons.

The relationship of cigarette smoking to lung cancer, the association of birth control pills with blood vessel problems, and the transmission patterns of AIDS all were identified in case-control studies that pointed the way for detailed, confirming investigations.

- *Cohort* or *incidence studies* are motion pictures. Researchers pick a group of people, or cohort (a cohort was a unit of a Roman legion). Then the researchers follow the people in the cohort over time, often for years, to see how some disease or diseases develop. These studies are costly and difficult. Subjects drop out or disappear. Large numbers must be studied to see rare events.

But cohort studies can be powerful instruments, and can substitute for randomized experiments that would be ethically impossible. You can't ethically expose a group to an agent that you suspect would cause a disease. You *can* watch a group so exposed.

Examples: The noted Framingham study of ways of life that might be associated with developing heart disease has followed more than 5,000 residents of that Massachusetts town since 1948. The American Cancer Society's 1952–55 study of 187,783 men aged 50 to 69, with 11,780 of them dying during that period, did much to establish that cigarette smoking was strongly associated with developing lung cancer.[11] Another method of classification, for both epidemiological and clinical studies, involves timing:

- **Retrospective studies** look back in time – at medical records, vital statistics, or people's recollections. People who have a disease are questioned to try to find common habits or exposures. Possible limitations to watch for: Memories may play tricks. Old records may be poor and misleading. Definitions of diseases and methods of diagnosis vary over the years. This is why attempts are underway to implement electronic health records, with standardized ways of recording diseases and treatments.
- **Prospective studies,** like the Framingham and the American Cancer Society studies, look forward. They focus sharply on a selected group who are all followed by the same statistical and medical techniques. For example, residents of the Gulf of Mexico and workers who helped clean up the oil in the water and on land will be followed for years to detect any deleterious health effects. And, having learned a lesson from the controversy over Gulf War Syndrome, the military is carefully following servicemen and -women who were deployed to Iraq to detect any unusual patterns of disease. (Note that the appropriate control group for this study is not drawn from the general population, but rather from servicemen and -women who were not sent to Iraq.)

Dr. Eugene Robin at Stanford tells how four separate retrospective clinical studies affirmed the accuracy of a test for blood clots in the lungs. When an adequate prospective clinical trial was done, most of the retrospective looks were proved wrong.[12]

- **Intervention studies** involve doing something to some of the subjects. The massive, hugely successful 1954 field trial of the Salk polio vaccine was a classic epidemiological intervention study – and a clinical trial too.[13] Another successful intervention study, a community trial, established the value of fluoridating water supplies to prevent tooth decay. Some towns had their water fluoridated; some did not. Blinding was impossible, but the striking difference in dental cavities that resulted was highly unlikely to have been caused by any placebo effect.

Writing about disease outbreaks

Epidemiologists study and act on other worrisome outbreaks that pop up regularly across the nation. These include serious respiratory ailments, various food-borne illnesses (with life-threatening *E. coli* just one example), and meningitis. They include the mosquito-borne West Nile virus that reached the United States from Africa in 1999 and continues to be an encephalitis threat, and all sorts of other diseases. And these disease detectives – just like police detectives – sometimes must move early, issuing warnings and alerts when very little evidence is in.

Dr. Michael Osterholm listed some things that reporters should keep in mind as they deal with the numbers while covering disease outbreaks:

1. **Common symptoms can inflate numbers.** When health officials investigate a food-borne outbreak, they can't assume that everyone who reports having symptoms actually has that illness.

   Diarrhea and gastrointestinal cramps are common and can be caused by a variety of things. Headaches and stiff necks can be caused by many things, not necessarily meningitis. Fever and aches can be caused by many things, not necessarily some new illness that's in the news. Legionnaires' disease can be confused with common forms of pneumonia.

   Health officials investigating an outbreak may classify cases into three groups: possible, probable, and confirmed. Reporters should report this and ask: How are you deciding which cases are in each group? Are lab tests needed to confirm the diagnosis?

2. **An increase in reported cases may be due to more reporting, not more actual cases.** When there are a lot of news reports about Lyme disease, or about food-borne outbreaks or whatever, more people are likely to see their doctors or phone public health agencies. Reported-case totals rise. The same number of cases may have been *occurring* before the news reports, although many were not being *reported*.

3. **What appears to be one big outbreak may be several mini-outbreaks.** Fortunately, epidemiologists often can use a relatively new technology, "genetic fingerprinting," to tell them whether scattered cases of an infectious illness are related.

   Example offered by Osterholm: An increased number of hepatitis A cases are being reported in a large metropolitan area. "Genetic fingerprinting" may show that the virus strains from all the cases are precisely the same, pointing to a single source of the outbreak. Or this lab test may show slight variations in the strains involved. Further study then may find that some of the cases started in a day-care center, some started with an infected food-handler, and some were introduced by a foreign traveler.

   So if there are scattered cases of some illnesses in your community with no clear link, ask if "genetic fingerprinting" is planned.

4. **When there's a national problem, check the numbers to see what's happening in your community.**

   Example: The nation's AIDS epidemic started with cases reported in California and New York. The virus got a chance to spread in those states before the peril was clearly recognized; for various reasons, the spread to and within other states has been uneven. The rates of AIDS cases (per 100,000 population) not only vary greatly from one state to another, but there often are big differences between metropolitan and rural areas.

   Other disease patterns vary from region to region, for a variety of reasons. All this may require different prevention priorities in different geographical areas, and different reporting by journalists.

   Epidemiological studies do have their limitations. They can link cigarette smoking to various types of cancer. But laboratory studies are needed to pin down just how smoking causes the cellular changes that spell malignancy. Epidemiological studies can show how a new type of virus is spreading and which parts of the population are most vulnerable. But laboratory studies and then clinical studies are needed to find a treatment or vaccine.

Despite this, the preventive messages that typically come out of epidemiological studies can be vitally important. And the associations discovered by epidemiological studies often point the way for the laboratory studies that must follow.

Example: "Epi studies" (as they often are called) first probed how AIDS was being spread, allowing the nation to take steps to limit that spread before the AIDS virus was even discovered.

And sometimes epidemiological studies provide evidence for the *absence* of something. Two examples: Thousands of women sued their doctors and several manufacturers of breast implants, claiming that silicone gel breast implants were causing their autoimmune disorders. Epidemiological studies showed that there was no association between the implants and the disorder. (By the way, animal studies also failed to show this toxicity.) And many parents sued pharmaceutical firms because they believed that anti-nausea medication taken during pregnancy caused tragic limb defects in their babies. Again, epidemiological studies showed that women who took this medication were no more likely to have babies with birth defects than women who didn't take the medication. However, despite these scientific findings, manufacturers pulled the drugs from the American market.

The "H1N1" Strain of Influenza

Epidemiologists also studied the 2009–10 pandemic (global epidemic) of a novel strain of H1N1 influenza. They found that while this "new flu" spread quickly and widely among people throughout the world, there was some welcome news as well. This strain didn't have an unusually high death rate, a problem that had characterized most earlier influenza pandemics. And surprisingly, unlike other influenza outbreaks, the elderly seemed less likely to get the flu, perhaps because they had lived through epidemics of an influenza with a similar but not identical "genetic fingerprint." And the epidemiologists' early detection of this new strain led to a relatively quick development of a vaccine, which helped reduce the toll even more.

Now some numbers:[14]

Depending on many variables and unknowns, an influenza pandemic could kill anywhere from about 200,000 to 2 million Americans, experts have estimated.

But the common strains of influenza that arrive every winter are no wimps. They kill, on average, about 36,000 Americans a year, according to the federal Centers for Disease Control and Prevention (visit cdc.gov). The aged and people with certain chronic illnesses are particularly vulnerable.[15]

To follow developments on the possibility of an influenza pandemic: click on pandemicflu.gov (U.S. government overview site); cdc.gov (federal Centers for Disease Control and Prevention; who.int (World Health Organization).

What's in a Name?

Many people call all sorts of minor stomach and other achy illnesses *"the flu."* But *influenza* is a specific respiratory illness that comes each winter. It can hit hard (and even kill some elderly and other vulnerable people), and may spread particularly quickly and widely.

Cancer is a collection of related diseases – all involving body cells that lose their normal control over growth. Even cancers of a specific body site (lung cancer, for example) have subtypes with different treatments and survival rates; hence the need for further development of personalized medicine approaches to treatment.

Hepatitis A is quite different from hepatitis B and C, and there are other types of hepatitis, too. And there are different types of diabetes, pneumonia, arthritis, heart disease, strokes, and other illnesses, each with their own treatment regimens and numbers.

Bottom line for journalists: Be clear about what you're writing about, and careful that the statistics match.

Notes

1. Jay A. Winsten, "Science and the Media; the Boundaries of Truth," *Health Affairs* (Spring 1985): 5–23.
2. C. Y. Wang et al., "Postexposure immunoprophylaxis of primary isolates by an antibody to HIV receptor complex," *Proceedings of the National Academy of Sciences, USA* 96 (1999): 10367–72.
3. Much of the discussion about disease outbreaks is based on an interview with Dr. Michael Osterholm, former Minnesota state epidemiologist and now director of the Center for Infectious Disease Research and Policy at the University of Minnesota.
4. Umberto Veronesi, "Cancer Research—Developing Better Clinical Trials," *Therapaeia* (May 1984): 31.

5. Deborah Zarin et al., "Issues in the Registration of Clinical Trials," *Journal of the American Medical Association* (May 16, 2007): 297.

6. See note 5.

7. Elie Dolgin, "Publication Bias Continues Despite Clinical-Trial Registration," http://www.nature.com/news/2009/090911/full/news.2009.902.html

8. Hooke, *How to Tell the Liars*.

9. http://www.cancer.gov/cancertopics/factsheet/therapy/herceptin/print

10. Bailar, "Science, Statistics."

11. E. Cuyler Hammond, "Smoking in Relation to Death Rates of One Million Men and Women" in *Epidemiological Approaches to the Study of Cancer and Other Chronic Diseases*, ed. W. Haenszel (Department of Health, Education and Welfare, National Cancer Institute Monograph no. 19, January 1986).

12. Eugene D. Robin, *Medical Care Can Be Hazardous to Your Health* (New York: Harper and Row, 1986).

13. Paul Meier, "The Biggest Public Health Experiment Ever," in *Statistics*, ed. Tanur et al.

14. Various news and other sources. The *New York Times* (March 28, 2006) devoted an entire Science Times section to an excellent report on avian influenza.

15. Ceci Connolly, "U.S. Plan for Flu Pandemic Revealed," *Washington Post*, April 16, 2006, and other news reports.

5

Your Questions
and Peer Review

Just because Dr. Famous or Dr. Bigshot says this is what he found doesn't mean it is necessarily so.

Dr. Arnold Relman, former editor of the
New England Journal of Medicine

Good questions can be golden.

One of this book's authors (Cohn) once asked Dr. Morris Fishbein, the provocative genius who long edited the *Journal of the American Medical Association*, "How can I, a reporter, tell whether a doctor is doing a good job of caring for his patients?" Fishbein immediately replied, "Ask him how often he has a patient take off his shirt."

His lesson was plain: No physical exam is complete unless the patient takes off his or her clothes.

Some top science journalists make it a habit to ask experts, at the end of an interview or a press conference, "What question should I have asked, but didn't?"

It's a double-win question. The interviewer gets a last crack at getting answers to questions that he or she forgot (or didn't know) to ask. The person being interviewed often appreciates the chance to say something that he or she has been thinking about. And gems often fall out of this final exchange.

News & Numbers: A Writer's Guide to Statistics, Third Edition. Victor Cohn and Lewis Cope with Deborah Cohn Runkle.
© 2012 Victor Cohn and Lewis Cope. Published 2012 by Blackwell Publishing Ltd.

Another type of example:

- Early in 1999 researchers reported on a big dietary study, involving about 89,000 women. Their key conclusion was that fiber in the diet doesn't lower the risk of colon cancer. *Time* magazine's Christine Gorman probed deeper for a bigger picture.

The result: The magazine's headline read "Still High on Fiber." While fiber may not protect against colon cancer, other studies provide strong evidence that it is "good for your heart" and helps to keep your body healthy in other ways, Gorman informed her readers.[1]

The lesson: Ask yourself, and ask others as necessary, "Do I have the full picture?"

In Chapter 3, we suggested that you ask researchers these basic questions about their conclusions or claims: How do you know? Have you (or others) done a study or any experiments? If so, were they acceptable ones, by general agreement? Were they without any substantial bias? Are the conclusions backed by believable statistical evidence? And what is the degree of certainty or uncertainty? How sure can you be?

And to put the study in perspective: Are your results fairly consistent with those from any related studies, and with general knowledge in the field? Have the findings resulted in a consensus among other experts in the field?

In some cases there may be no studies at all, only anecdotal information that raises some concern. "There are four cases in our block" may be worth investigating, maybe worth even a cautious news story, but there is not yet anything close to certainty.

Assuming that there has been a study, a researcher's scientific presentation may answer all of these questions to your satisfaction. In fact, if you must ask too many questions, that in itself might hint that the study is lacking in some regard.

But some studies, some claims, some controversies require you to probe deeper. You may need to focus on one specific area, or several.

Don't be reticent about asking what you need to know. You're just following the path of good science. A properly skeptical scientist, starting a study, may begin with a *null hypothesis* – that a new treatment *won't* work. Then the scientist sees whether or not the evidence disproves the null hypothesis – and, in doing so, demonstrates that there is statistically significant evidence that the new treatment really works.

This approach is much like the law's presumption of innocence. It is for the prosecutor to prove beyond reasonable doubt that the suspect is guilty. A journalist, without being cynical, should be equally skeptical and greet every claim by saying, in words or thought, "Show me."

Start the Smorgasbord

This chapter contains a smorgasbord of questions. Like any good smorgasbord, pick and choose what you want and need. And, of course, you can fashion questions of your own.[2]

1. Is the study large enough to pass statistical muster?

How many subjects (patients, cases, observations, etc.) are you talking about? Are these numbers large enough, statistically rigorous enough, to get the answers you want? Was there an adequate number of patients to show a difference between treatments?

Small numbers can sometimes carry weight. "Sometimes small samples are the best we can do," one researcher says. But larger numbers are always more likely to pass statistical muster.

The number can depend on the situation. A thorough physiological study of five cases of some difficult disorder may be important. One new case of smallpox would be a shocker in a world in which smallpox has supposedly been eliminated. In June 1981, the federal Centers for Disease Control and Prevention reported that five young men, all active homosexuals, had been treated for the uncommon disease *Pneumocystis carinii* pneumonia at three Los Angeles hospitals.[3] This alerted the world to what became the AIDS epidemic.

P **(for probability) value** – Could your results have occurred just by chance? Have any statistical tests been applied to test this?

Did you calculate a *P* value? Was it favorable – .05 or less? *P* values and confidence statements need not be regarded as straitjackets, but like jury verdicts, they indicate reasonable doubt or reasonable certainty.

Remember that positive findings are more likely to be reported and published than negative findings. Remember that a favorable-sounding *P* value of .05 means only that there is just 1 chance in 20, or a 5 percent probability, that the statistics could have come out this way by pure chance when there was actually no effect.

There are ways and ways of arriving at *P* values. For example, an investigator may choose to report one of several end points: death, length of survival, blood pressure, other measurements, or just the patient's condition on leaving the hospital. All can be important, but a *P* value can be misleading if the wrong one is picked or emphasized. In cancer studies, different metrics are used; sometimes *survival time* is reported and sometimes the study looks at *progression-free survival time*. Be sure to ask what metric was used.

You might ask yourself: How important is hospital discharge if many of the patients die within a few days after returning home?

A general question you might ask researchers: Did you collaborate with a statistician in both your design and your analysis?

2. Is the study designed well? Could unintentional bias have affected the results?

Type and design of study – What kind of study was it? Do you think it was the right kind of study to get the answer you sought?

Was there a systematic research plan or design? And a *protocol* (a set of rules for the study)? Was the design drawn before you started your study? What specific questions or hypotheses did you set out to test or answer? Why did you do it that way?

If an investigator patiently tells you about an acceptable-sounding design, that's worth a brownie point. If the answer is "Huh?" or a nasty one, that may tell you something else. (See Chapter 4 for a discussion of study types and their uses and limits.)

Patient selection – Who were your subjects? How were they selected? What were your criteria for admission to the study? Were rigorous laboratory tests used (if possible) to define the patients' diagnoses?

Was the assignment of subjects to treatment or a comparison group done on a random basis? Were the patients admitted to the study before the randomization? This helps eliminate bias.

If the subjects weren't randomized, why not? One statistician says, "If it is a non-randomized study, a biased investigator can get some extraordinary results by carefully picking his subjects."

Control group – Was there a control or comparison group? If not, the study will be weaker. Who or what were your controls or bases for comparison? In other words: When you say you have such and such a result, what are you comparing it with? Are the study or patient group and the control group similar in all respects, except for the treatment or other variable being studied?

Thomas M. Vogt calls "comparison of noncomparable groups probably ... the single most common error in the medical and popular literature on health and disease."[4]

Representative? – Were your patients and controls representative of the general population? Or of a particular population – people with the disease or condition you are interested in?

The answers here go a long way toward answering these questions: To what populations are the results applicable? Would the association hold for other groups?

If your groups are not comparable to the general population or some important populations, have you taken steps to adjust for this? Have you used either statistical adjustment or stratification of your sample to find out about specific groups? Or both? Samples can be adjusted for age, for example, to make an older- or younger-than-average sample more nearly comparable to the general populace.

"Blinding" and quality control – Was the study blinded? In a study comparing drugs or other forms of treatment with a placebo or dummy treatment, did (1) those administering the treatment, (2) those getting it, and (3) those assessing the outcome know who was getting what? Or were they indeed blinded, and not know who was getting what?

Could those giving or getting the treatment have easily guessed which was which by a difference in some physical reaction?

Not every study can be a blind study. One researcher says, "There can be ethical problems in not telling patients what drug they're taking and the possible side effects. People are not guinea pigs." True, but a blinded study will always carry more conviction.

Were there other accepted quality controls – for example, making sure (perhaps by counting pills or studying urine samples) that the patients who were supposed to take a pill really took it? Were you able to follow your study plan?

Surveys, questionnaires, interviews – Were the questions likely to elicit accurate, reliable answers? Respondents' answers can differ sharply, depending on how questions are asked.

Example: In one study, 1,153 people were asked: Which is safer – a treatment that kills 10 percent of every 100 patients or a treatment with a 90 percent survival rate? More people voted for the second way of saying precisely the same thing.[5]

People commonly give inaccurate answers to sensitive questions, such as those about sexual behavior. They are notoriously inaccurate in reporting their own medical histories, even those of recent months. And they may fudge their answers when asked if they do things they know they should, such as using the car's seatbelts.

Dropouts – How many of your study subjects completed the study? Do you account for those who dropped out and tell why they did? Were the dropouts different in some way from the other subjects in the study?

Every study has dropouts. Dr. David Sackett at McMaster University says, "Patients do not disappear ... for trivial reasons. Rather, they leave ... because they refuse therapy, recover, die, or retire to the Sunbelt with their permanent disability."

If an investigator ignores those who didn't do well and dropped out, it can make the outcome look better. Sometimes those who died of "other causes" are listed among "survivors" of the disease being investigated. This is sometimes done on the theory that, after all, they didn't die of the target cause. But this can make a treatment look better than it really is, unless there are equal numbers of such deaths in every branch of the study. Likewise, it is equally misleading to say a cancer patient had only a one-month survival time following treatment if the patient died in a car accident. There are statistical methods for accounting for these circumstances. Were they used?

Sackett adds, "The loss to follow-up of 10 percent of the original inception cohort is cause for concern. If 20 percent or more are not accounted for, the results ... are probably not worth reading."[6] (Vogt comments on this: "Generally true, but utterly dependent on the situation.")

Potential conflict of interest – Ask, when appropriate: Where did the money to support the study come from? Many honest investigators are financed by companies that may profit from the outcome. All studies are financed by some source. In any case, the public should know any pertinent connections.

3. Did the study last long enough?

How long was the study's follow-up? Was it long enough to see whether the drug or other treatment can provide long-term benefits? How long do patients ordinarily survive with this disease? Were your patients followed long enough to really know the outcomes, good or bad?

Example: A new drug may put some cancer patients into remission – but it will take more time to see if the drug will lengthen survival. Many studies with these limitations still should be reported, but the limitations should be noted.

There are equally important questions about the length of some nonmedical studies.

Our weather, by its very nature, has a lot of ups and downs. Some days are rainy, some dry. We'll always have occasional super-cold-snap winters in the mix of things. Climate looks at the big, long-term picture – the averages and trends. It takes decades – or more – of data to discern major climate shifts. Most experts – but not all – now agree that global warming is real and is linked to the burning of fossil fuels. A key debate now is over how urgent the threat might be and what needs to be done about it.

4. Are there other possible explanations for the findings? Any other reasons to question the conclusions?

Cause-and-effect? – Remember that association is not necessarily causation. A virus found in patients with a particular illness may not be the cause of that illness. A chemical found in the water supply may not be the cause of people's ailments.

Always "view mathematical associations with a healthy degree of skepticism," cautions Dr. Michael Greenberg at Rutgers.

Yet, with care, researchers can build a case. A good experiment, controlling all variables, can sometimes demonstrate cause and effect almost surely. A strong association coupled with lab or animal studies may be persuasive. In other cases, proof may be more elusive.

But when does a close association in an observational study (rather than a controlled experiment) indicate causation? There are several possible criteria that you can ask about while discussing the overall picture with a researcher:

- Is the association statistically strong (like the association between smoking and lung cancer)?
- Does the supposed cause precede the effect?
- Do high doses of a chemical (or something else) tend to cause more problems than lower doses? Heavy smokers are indeed at greater risk than moderate smokers, and moderate smokers at greater risk than light smokers. (With some things, there may a threshold effect, an effect only after some minimum dose.)
- Is the association consistent when different research methods are used?
- Does the association make biological sense? Does it agree with current biological and physiological knowledge? You can't follow this test out the window. Much biological fact is ill understood. Also, Harvard's Mosteller warns, "*Someone* nearly always will claim to see a [biological or physiological] association. But the people who know the most may not be willing to."[7]
- Did you look for other explanations – confounders, or confounding variables, that may be producing or helping produce the association?

Sometimes we read that married people live longer than singles. Does marriage really increase life expectancy, or may medical or other problems make some people less likely to marry and also die sooner? Maybe the Dutch thought that storks brought babies because better-off families had more chimneys, more storks, and more babies. (See "Bias and Alternate Explanations" in Chapter 3 for more examples.)

Does a treatment really work? – Could the improvement in the patients' condition be due to something other than the new treatment they are receiving? Some questions to probe for other possible explanations:

Could the patients' improvements be changes that are occurring in the normal course of their disease? Some medical problems (multiple sclerosis, some forms of arthritis, etc.) have symptoms that tend to wax and wane; improvements may be due to the normal course of the illness rather than a new treatment being studied.

Could an old treatment that a patient received before the new one be responsible for a delayed improvement? Or, if a patient is receiving more than one treatment, which one is responsible for the improvement? Or might both be helping? When studying some alternative therapy, ask: Was the patient also receiving some conventional treatment that might have been responsible for the improvement?

If a treatment appears to work against one type of diabetes or pneumonia or heart problem or whatever, are you assuming that this will work against other types of that illness? What is the basis for that assumption? This is a particularly important area to probe in cancer treatments, where, for example, a treatment might help for one form of lung cancer, but not for other forms of lung cancer.

If all the patients in a study had an early or a mild form of an illness, you may need to ask the researcher: Why do you think your treatment will help patients with advanced or severe cases? But the reverse also can be true. Hospital populations and "worst cases" are not necessarily typical of patients in general. And often experimental treatments are tried first on the desperately or hopelessly ill, just to see if there is any effect at all. This method avoids testing a possibly toxic new treatment on individuals who otherwise might recover or for whom a standard treatment is available. But will a treatment tested on the sickest of the sick work on those in less dire straits? Be on guard against any improper generalizations.

Even claims for medications that reduce symptoms of some minor ailments need to be questioned. Doctors often say, "Most things are better in the morning," and they're often right when it comes to minor aches

61

and pains that tend to wax and wane. So: Is the patient feeling better because of the medications, or simply because of the tincture of time?

Careful design of the study and analysis of the data can help get at the answers for many of these questions and others as well.

Measuring what works – How did you know or decide when your patients were cured or improved? Were there explicit, objective outcome criteria? That is, were there firm measurements or test results rather than physicians' observations in interviews, physical examinations, or chart reviews – all techniques highly subject to great observer variation and inaccuracy?

In studies of improvement or relief from pain, which in some cases is a hard-to-quantify outcome, ask: Was there some systematic way of making an assessment? Scales have been developed to assess and quantify the subjective experience of pain. Were they used? (When even a single patient says that she or he feels relief from pain, that's important for that patient. But only a careful study can make a judgment about whether a pain-relief technique is likely to help other patients as well.)

If two or more groups were compared for survival: Were they judged by the same disease definitions at the start, and the same measures of severity and outcome?

Looking for the bottom line – Did the intervention have the good results that were intended? Has there been an evaluation to see whether they were useful results?

Investigators often report that a drug or other measure has lowered cholesterol levels in the blood. Good. But were the investigators able to show that this particular method of cholesterol reduction cut the number of heart attacks? Or cut the mortality rate? Or was the reduction of a supposed risk factor itself taken to mean the hoped-for outcome?

In such cases, the cholesterol reading (or other lab findings) is called a *marker* or *surrogate* or *proxy*. If a new treatment lowers cholesterol levels in the blood, the researcher hopes that this means it also will reduce the risk of heart attacks. But that bottom-line answer can take time.

Questions that the journalist can ask the researcher (and sometimes other experts): Is a particular lab test a reliable predictor of final outcome? What's the evidence for that? What follow-up studies may be needed to get a conclusive answer?

Also watch out for unexpected effects and side effects of treatments. An investigator reported that when women with heart disease took statins, heart-related deaths went down, but the drugs didn't reduce the overall death rate. Further, in otherwise-healthy women taking statins to lower their cholesterol, there is little evidence that the drug reduces the risk of heart disease. And some evidence shows that women are more likely than men to suffer serious side effects from this class of drugs.[8]

Another example of an area in which reporters need to keep their eyes on the bottom line: Public health officials may announce that, in a screening campaign, 200 people were found to have high blood pressure and were referred to their doctors. But how many then went to their doctors? How many of those received optimum treatment? Were their blood pressures reduced? (If they were, the evidence is strong that they should suffer fewer strokes.)

Did you really do any good? To whom do your results apply? Can they be generalized to a larger population? Are your patients like the average doctor's patients? Often, medical studies are conducted at academic health centers. How will the treatments work in a rural or inner-city setting? Is there any basis in these findings for any patient to ask his or her doctor for a change in treatment? Clinic populations, hospital populations, and the "worst cases" are not necessarily typical of patients in general, and improper generalization is unfortunately common in the medical literature.

Finding what breakdowns can reveal – Did you do a stratified analysis – a breakdown of the data by strata such as gender, ethnicity, socioeconomic status, geographical area, occupation?

A treatment may work better for women than for men, or vice versa (see the statin example above). Some people are more vulnerable to a particular disease than are others. Men commonly have more cirrhosis of the liver than women because they drink more. More women than men die each year from heart disease. And cancer is the leading cause of death for people under age 85.[9] Stratification helps in all such studies.

5. Do the conclusions fit other evidence?

Are your results consistent with other experimental findings and knowledge in the field? If not, why? Have your results been repeated or confirmed or supported by other studies?

Virtually no single study proves anything. Consistency of results among human trials, animal experiments, and laboratory tests is a good start. Two or more studies in humans can build even more confidence.

One scientist warns, however, "You have to be wary about a grab bag of studies with different populations and different circumstances." To this Mosteller adds, "Yes, be wary, but consistency across such differences cheers me up."

Meta-analysis is the statistical analysis of several low-power research studies to integrate the results. In effect, it adds several studies together to try to come up with stronger conclusions. The trick is to make sure that the researcher adds only apples to apples. Dr. John Bailar tells us that, despite possible pitfalls, "meta-analysis of several low-power reports *may* come to stronger conclusions than any one of them alone" [italics ours].[10]

6. Do I have the full picture? What about side effects, cost issues, and ethical concerns?

Are there important side effects from a new drug (or other new treatment) being studied? Any other problems? Do the potential benefits outweigh these problems?

If it's a weight-loss or other type of diet, is it reasonable to expect that people will follow your diet?

Have any ethical problems arisen during the research? Do you see any ethical problems ahead?

What would the new treatment (or whatever) cost? Do the potential benefits outweigh the costs?

Example of a costs–benefits debate: In the summer of 1999, the U.S. Food and Drug Administration approved a new inhaled drug to treat influenza, overruling a panel of advisers who had concluded that the new drug was only marginally effective. But in the United Kingdom – the home base of the drug's maker, Glaxo Wellcome PLC – the government-run National Health Service ordered physicians not to prescribe the drug, after an advisory group there concluded that the costs "would be disproportionate to the benefits obtained by influenza sufferers."[11]

Others' Views and Peer Review

7. What do other experts say? Has there been formal peer review?

Ask the researcher: Who disagrees with you? And why?

Ask others in the same field: How do other informed people regard this report – and these investigators? Are they speaking in their own area of expertise, or have they shown real mastery if they have ventured outside it? Have their past results generally held up? And what are some good questions I can ask them? True, a lot of brilliant and original work has been pooh-poohed for a time by others. Still, scientists survive only by eventually convincing their colleagues.

Has there been a review of the data and conclusions by any disinterested parties?

Medicine and health – Have the study and its findings been examined by peer-review referees who were sent the article by a journal editor? Has the work been published or accepted by a reputable journal? If not, why not?

Medical meetings also are an important source of news. But research papers presented at meetings normally have not been reviewed with the rigor used by good medical journals to select the papers that they publish. So reporters may need to ask more questions or, if they attend the meeting, listen to what other experts at the session say.

Some free-circulation journals and medical magazines, supported totally by advertising, print summary articles rather than original research reports. These articles normally are not as rigorously screened as those published in the traditional journals. They may make news too, but the limits on their peer-review process should be kept in mind.

Other fields – Peer-reviewed journal articles and meetings also are important sources of news in other fields, ranging from economics to crime prevention.

But many people outside academia do studies in various nonhealth fields, and these studies may never be sent to journals or be presented at major meetings. Many good economics reports and environmental studies fit into this category.

It's still fair to ask these researchers whether their conclusions have been checked by independent experts. The answers may help you determine how deeply you want to probe with other questions.

Top journals – In science as a whole, including biology and other basic medical sciences, *Science* and the British *Nature* are indispensable.

In general medicine and clinical science at the physician's level, the most useful journals include (but aren't limited to) the *New England Journal of Medicine*, the *Journal of the American Medical Association*, and the British *Lancet*.

In epidemiology, a good source, among others, is the *American Journal of Epidemiology*. Some important epidemiological studies are reported in the *New England Journal of Medicine* and other clinically oriented journals.

There are many equally good medical specialty journals, as well as mediocre ones. Ask people in any field: What are the most reliable journals, those where you would want your work published?

Warning label – Peer review can't provide a guarantee. Even the best of journals can print clinkers sometimes.

"Scientific journals are records of work, not of revealed truth," says the *New England Journal of Medicine*'s Dr. Arnold Relman.[12]

Journalistic Perspective

8. What now?

Now we get to some bottom-line journalistic questions that can help put everything in perspective. *Ask researchers, as needed:*

- What do you think should happen next?
- What are your plans?
- What steps lie ahead before this can benefit people?
- How long should this take?
- What is the potential?
- How confident are you?
- What could go wrong?
- Are other researchers working on approaches that are different from yours?
- How do you feel about the future of your research?

Getting Down to the Writing ...

As you prepare to write, consider: Do the conclusions make good sense to me? Do the data really justify the conclusions? If the researcher has extrapolated beyond the evidence, has he or she explained why and made sense?

Does the researcher frankly document or discuss the possible biases and flaws in the study? It's a big plus for one who does. Does the researcher admit that the conclusion may be tentative or equivocal? Dr. Robert Boruch at Northwestern University says, "It requires audacity and some courage to say, 'I don't know.'"[13]

Does the author disclose potential conflicts of interest?

Read the journal article yourself, if there is one. Too many news releases tout articles that read far more conservatively than the PR version. Ask the researcher for a copy. Or check the Internet, where some journals' articles are posted. Or check online at plos.org (Public Library of Science). Or look for it at a hospital's or medical school's library.

Do the authors use qualifying phrases? If such phrases are important, reporters should share them with their readers or viewers.

"What proportion of papers will satisfy [all] the requirements for scientific proof and clinical applicability?" Sackett writes. "Not very many ... After all, there are only a handful of ways to do a study properly but a thousand ways to do it wrong."[14]

Despite impeccable design, some studies yield answers that turn out to be wrong. Some fail for lack of understanding of physiology and disease. Even the soundest studies may provoke controversy. In particular, some "may meet considerable resistance when they discredit the only treatment currently available," Sackett says.

Journalists need to tread a narrow path between believing everything and believing nothing. Also – we are journalists – some of the controversies make good stories.

Special Situations

"Hindsight bias" – As with much of life, it's easier to see some problems in retrospect. After a study is completed, reporters may see how a study could have been better designed to find more answers. Journalists should ask themselves: Should the researcher have been able to foresee the problem at the start of the study? Or did the researcher simply overlook something that any researcher might have overlooked?

The answers should determine how the journalist reports the study's limitations. And sometimes this should be done gently, pointing out the everyday comparison with seeing things in hindsight.

Basic research – Some genetics, cell-function, and other research is at such a basic level that researchers say they don't know how their findings could be put to use. Reporters should realize that such findings can be important building blocks for later scientific advances.

The Art of Interviewing

Six simple questions can do super jobs:[15]

1. To break down the complex: **"How do you explain this to your wife (or husband, or children, or neighbors)?"**
2. The single word that can often clarify, and also offer breadth to many stories: **"Why?"**

3. To probe: **"Who are your critics? What do they say?"**
4. Bottom line: **"What's the key significance of your findings to patients (or the public)?"**
5. To get a colorful, human touch for your article: **"How did you feel when you reached that eureka moment (or other key point in your research)?" "Were you surprised by the result?"**
6. At the end of an interview or press conference: **"What's the question that I should have asked but didn't?"**

Notes

1. Christine Gorman, "Still High on Fiber," *Time*, February 1, 1999.
2. Many of these questions are, in our view, common sense. But Frederick Mosteller differs with us on use of that term. If something is a common sense idea, he says, "surely all would have thought of it. So it must be uncommon sense after all." He makes good sense.
3. *Morbidity and Mortality Weekly Report* (Centers for Disease Control and Prevention, Atlanta) 30 (June 1981): 250–52.
4. Vogt, *Making Health Decisions*.
5. Barbara McNeil et al., "On the Elicitation of Preferences for Alternative Therapies," *New England Journal of Medicine* 306, no. 21 (May 27, 1982): 1259–62.
6. David Sackett in *Coping*, ed. Warren.
7. Mosteller talk at CASW seminar.
8. Catherine Elton, "Do Statins Work Equally for Men and Women?" *Time* (March 29, 2010).
9. http://www.benbest.com/lifeext/causes.html
10. Bailar, "Science, Statistics."
11. Various news reports, including *Wall Street Journal*, October 11, 1999.
12. Arnold Relman in *Clinical Trials*, ed. Shapiro and Louis.
13. Robert Boruch, quoted in "Taking the Measure, or Mismeasure, of It All," *New York Times*, August 28, 1984.
14. Sackett in *Clinical Trials*, ed. Shapiro and Louis.
15. Sources: expert-interviewers who spoke at a National Association of Science Writers symposium; the book's authors; other journalists.

Part II

Now Down to Specifics

A Guide to Part II of
News & Numbers

The first five chapters covered the basics. Now to specific areas:

6. **Tests and Drug Trials**
   Measuring what health care is needed and what works.

7. **Vital Statistics**
   Measuring life and health, with a detailed look at cancer numbers.

8. **Health Costs, Quality, and Insurance**
   Measuring the quality of health plans and hospitals, and all health care costs.

9. **Our Environment**
   Measuring harms and concerns, including a look at the limitations of science.

10. **Writing About Risks**
    This new chapter ties together, and adds much to, the discussion of risks throughout the book.

11. **Polls**
    Measuring public opinion with polls and surveys, plus a look at focus groups and "snowball sampling."

12. **Statistical Savvy for Many Types of News**
    Reporting newsy numbers in many fields, plus a look at some missing numbers.

6

Tests and Drug Trials

Ask to see the numbers, not just the pretty colors.
Dr. Richard Margolin, National Institutes of Health,
describing PET scans to reporters

It's important for physicians to know how much faith they can place in various medical tests, because an increasing amount of medical care is based on the results of these tests – lab tests, imaging studies, and more. It's also important for medical journalists to have a feel for the special questions they need to ask about such tests. Let's start with some real-life examples that illustrate key principles:

Cost considerations about medical tests aren't limited to the fees charged for the tests. Some good tests can save money, through improved care and by eliminating some unnecessary care.

A good example: In 2006, the federal Medicare program decided to start paying for a $400 test designed to help determine if a patient is a good candidate for an implanted cardiac defibrillator. Once implanted, the defibrillator can send an electrical shock if the heart stops working, and this often can restore a normal heartbeat. These defibrillators cost about $30,000 each, so the test may save a lot of money by eliminating the use of these implants in patients who are not likely to benefit – not to mention sparing many patients from the surgeons' scalpels.[1]

News & Numbers: A Writer's Guide to Statistics, Third Edition. Victor Cohn and Lewis Cope with Deborah Cohn Runkle.
© 2012 Victor Cohn and Lewis Cope. Published 2012 by Blackwell Publishing Ltd.

Genetic tests: **Getting the right drug to the right patient** is becoming a major goal of medical research and practice, particularly in the treatment of cancer. This targeted approach to cancer care comes under the heading of *personalized medicine* and is beginning to redefine traditional treatment methods.

Scientists have discovered that cancer tumors can be characterized by their genetics. And even tumors from the same location can have very different genetic markers, which leads medical researchers to devise treatments that target the genetic pathways particular to that kind of tumor. What this means is that two patients with, say, breast or colon cancers may receive very different treatments for their cancer. The Food and Drug Administration (FDA) has issued guidance to doctors that advises them to test some tumors for genetic markers and treat appropriately.

One example: Physicians are using a molecular genetic test to detect an excess of the HER2 protein on the surface of breast cancer tumors. Women with too much HER2 do not usually respond positively to standard treatments. But now their doctors can prescribe the gene-based drug Herceptin, which binds to the protein and deactivates it. This test and the right treatment have been shown to increase survival by 33 percent and reduce recurrence by 50 percent.[2]

Another example: The KRAS colon cancer test identifies patients with a normal gene called KRAS. These patients respond well to a drug called cetuximab. However, about 40 percent of colon cancer patients have a mutated form of the gene and do not respond to the drug. In fact, if they get the drug they are at risk for damaging side effects. This test allows doctors to prescribe the right treatment.[3]

These examples also mean that expensive and risky treatments will not be tried on patients who are highly unlikely to respond positively, possibly a money-saver in these cost-conscious times.

Alan Mertz, American Clinical Laboratory Association President, says that "In many ways, genetic testing represents the future of cancer care."

The mammography controversy: Cost not a factor? In 2009, a controversy erupted regarding the frequency at which women should receive routine mammography screening for breast cancer. After reviewing many studies, the federal government's Preventive Services Task Force reversed earlier advice by recommending that those women ages 40 to 49 who are not at elevated risk for breast cancer forgo routine mammography and that similarly situated women ages 50 to 59 should be screened once every two years, instead of the previously recommended yearly tests. Some critics claimed that the new recommendations were based on cost considerations, but Dr. Diana Petitti, vice chairman of the task force, denied this. She said that the benefits of routine mammography – how many cancers are detected – were weighed against the risks – how many false positives popped up, how many unnecessary follow-up tests were performed, and how much radiation women were exposed to in following up on the false positives.

But the American Cancer Society and the American College of Obstetrics and Gynecology stood by the old guidelines. The immediate result: Doctors' offices began receiving calls from patients wondering what they should do, and Dr. Susan Boolbol, the chief of breast cancer surgery at Beth Israel Medical Center in New York, said that the number of "no-shows" at the breast imaging department doubled. Whether these new guidelines change women's (and doctors') behavior in the long run remains to be seen.[4]

This chapter also covers the testing of new drug treatments before they can be put onto the market for widespread use, and how animals serve as stand-ins for us. But we'll first look at …

Medical Tests for Patients

A good test should detect both health and disease, and do so with high accuracy. The measures of the value of a clinical test – one used for medical diagnosis – are sensitivity and specificity, or simply the ability to avoid false negatives and false positives.

Sensitivity is how well a test identifies a disease or condition in those who have it. Sensitive tests miss few, if any, cases of the disease. Those missed cases are called *false negatives*.

Example: If 100 people with an illness are tested and 90 test positive, the test's sensitivity is 90 percent.

Specificity is how well a test identifies those who do *not* have the disease or condition. It is how well the test avoids *false positives*, or mistaken identifications.

Example: If 100 healthy people are tested and 90 test negative, the test's specificity is 90 percent.

In a nutshell: Sensitivity tells us about disease present. Specificity tells us about disease absent.

If the terms were used with home burglar alarms, sensitivity would reflect how well the system will detect an actual burglar. Specificity would reflect how prone the system is to false alarms.

Almost every test produces some false positives and some false negatives, and the two qualities are inversely related. The more sensitive you make a test to try to find every case, the less specific it will be and the more false positives you will get. The more specific you make it to try to avoid false labeling, the less sensitive it will be and the more false negatives you will get.

Testing the tests

The main questions that a reporter needs to ask the person who unveils a new test for AIDS or cancer or diabetes are: How many false negatives and false positives do you get? How do you know this? Have you done an adequate trial?

A new test should be tried and assessed by blinded observers in subjects chosen, by some definitive diagnosis, as patients who have the condition being sought. (This diagnosis may be by surgery, biopsy, long-term follow-up, or some other precise method.)

The new test should be tried as well in healthy people, and often it should also be tried in some people who have a condition frequently confused with the one being studied.

How well should a test do in avoiding false negatives and false positives? That may depend on its goal.

If the main aim is not to miss some serious condition, the test may shoot for high sensitivity to pick up every possible case and accept the false positives.

If the main concern is avoiding false positives in a disease doctors can't do much about anyway, or if the treatment itself carries significant danger, one may opt for more specificity.

Examples of the importance of sensitivity: Doubt was expressed about some tests for strep throat, because in 25 reports their sensitivity ranged from a reasonably acceptable 93 percent to an unacceptably low 65 percent. In short, there were too many false negatives for this illness.

A study group evaluated one firm's home pregnancy-testing kits whose maker claimed they detected pregnancy 95 to 98 percent of the time. Testing them in 144 pregnant women, the study group found them only 75.6 percent sensitive – one false negative in every four tests.[5]

Nevertheless, researchers sometimes have to accept poor sensitivity in a test for a particular disease, if it's the best they can do. A poor test may be better than no test.

Other potential questions about the testing of tests:

- Is this the right test for this particular condition? Epidemiologist Gary Friedman offered this example: Measuring a heart rate by putting your fingers on someone's wrist (taking a radial pulse) would lack validity for some patients with certain disturbances in heart rhythm, because some of their heartbeats produce too weak a pulse to be felt at the wrist.[6]
- How reliable, or reproducible, is the test? Does a series of observations produce the same or nearly the same result? If the results of a test typically vary, it must be repeated, perhaps several times, to get a mean (average) and a more reliable result.

But you should recognize that some results may vary through no fault of the test. For example, your blood pressure may be different when you are relaxed and when you are tense, or at different times of the day.

All tests are subject to error. Results can be affected by diet, drugs, exposure of a blood sample to light, a malfunctioning instrument, or a cockeyed observer.

There are some test results that don't have numbers. These include such things as listening for heart murmurs. Although trained people do these tests well, there can be more room for subjective judgments and differing opinions.

The lesson, if you're a patient or are writing about patients: Be cautious about letting yourself (or anyone else) be sentenced to a dire diagnosis on the basis of any one test. Still, one bone-marrow examination may indicate leukemia; one X-ray may clearly show a fracture.

- What's normal? There is also a potential trap in the word "normal." Some testers use it to mean average or statistically typical. Others use it to mean healthy or desirable or free of disease. "Within the normal range," a phrase often used, can mean little unless explained.

Example: Someone tells you that your serum cholesterol – the amount of cholesterol in your blood – is 210 (milligrams per deciliter) and that's not much above average for adult Americans. But it is too high to be optimal in the view of physicians who think it's associated with an elevated risk of atherosclerosis, or clogged arteries.

Similarly, "abnormal" may just mean that a particular laboratory finds that you're in the top or bottom 5 or 10 percent of test results at that lab or some group of labs. Thus "abnormal" might or might not mean anything clinically, and you may be perfectly healthy.

Ask: Does "normal" mean average, or does it mean okay? Does "abnormal" mean atypical, or unhealthy?

- Can any test find the answer? Few tests, however negative the result, are sure enough to give us a "clean bill of health."

Example: In January 1987, a usually excellent radio news program said tests on President Reagan had ruled out any spread of his earlier cancer. But cancer's spread is often undetectable and therefore unmeasurable, though it may later manifest itself. Such tests could only show that no spread of cancer had been found. In assessing health or disease, a good physician considers the results of a combination of several tests, if possible, as well as physical signs, symptoms, your behavior, and your history.

Screening tests

In addition to clinical tests to investigate some complaint, there are screening tests of normal persons, designed to pick out those who might have some condition but need further examination to confirm it.

Examples: routine Pap tests, mammograms, the tuberculin test to find those exposed to the TB bacillus, multiphasic testing for many conditions.

Keep in mind:

- A screening test should not be so rough that it exposes hundreds or thousands of actually healthy people to worry and expense, to possibly harmful further testing by chemical or invasive means, or to possibly harmful surgery or other treatment. This is especially true of the hundreds of new genetic tests that are being developed. Many of these tests are marketed DTC (Direct to Consumer), meaning that they are ordered by consumers, not doctors. If the results tell consumers they are at "high risk" for some disease or other, they might consult their physicians who, having little knowledge of how to interpret these tests, will send their patients on to higher-priced specialists or for further, perhaps unnecessary, tests.
- Studies that try to assess screening tests can be deceiving. People who take better care of themselves – or, perversely, those most likely to have the disease – may self-select themselves as test subjects. Again, new genetic tests are often developed by screening large numbers of people with a certain disease.

These tests need to be validated on an even larger population selected at random.

• Many authorities think society should forgo screening programs unless a test of demonstrated value attacks an important health problem that doctors can do something about, at a cost within reason, or if risk of a future disease can be lessened by changes in behavior or by taking a medication. However, insurers are reluctant to reimburse for tests that have no proven clinical usefulness.

A cancer test and a new vaccine – As noted in Chapter 2, medical recommendations often need to be updated as new knowledge is gained.

Case history of the Pap test: Until 1980, the American Cancer Society recommended that women have an annual Pap test to detect early signs that cervical cancer might be developing. The guidelines now allow up to three years between testing for many women after a series of normal findings.[7] Statistical studies concluded that this would be equally effective in detecting the problem at an easy-to-treat stage.

And in 2006, the FDA approved a vaccine to protect against two types of the human papilloma virus (HPV) that are responsible for about 70 percent of all cervical cancer. But because the vaccine "will not provide protection against all of the types of HPV that can cause cervical cancer, women will still need Pap tests," the cancer society says. Still, some experts speculate that the vaccine, approved for use in females ages 9 through 26, may bring some reduction in the frequency of Pap testing down the road.[8]

Pap test details: For information of how age and some other factors can affect Pap testing recommendations for some patients, click on the Cancer Society's web site at cancer.org.

Cost considerations – In writing about costs, consider not only how much the screening test itself will cost, but how much will be spent on follow-up tests to eliminate false positives. This may be particularly important for early-detection tests for colon and prostate cancer, research indicates. But remember the life-saving potentials, too.[9]

Drugs and Drug Trials

Many authorities recommend mistrusting any doctor who says, "Don't worry. I've been using this drug for years, and I've never seen these adverse reactions you read about." For starters, this physician may not be seeing the types of patients most vulnerable (by age, race, etc.) to side effects. But even more important, no single doctor can be seeing enough patients to make sweeping claims about safety.

By one calculation, "the individual physician is in a functional sense 'blind' to treatment-related risk" that occurs any less commonly than once in about 200 patients.[10] Drugs have been withdrawn or forced into restricted use because of adverse reactions in the range of 1 in 1,000 to 1 in 30,000. So if a doctor has treated only 200 patients with the drug, it is highly likely he will not have seen any adverse reactions. In other words, his relatively small sample lacks the *power* discussed in Chapter 3.

Are such drug withdrawals good or bad for society and for patients? The Food and Drug Administration, which evaluates drugs, is alternately attacked as the protector of venal drug companies foisting harmful drugs on the public, and as the citadel of needless regulation that denies good drugs to patients and profits to businesses.

The best course is not always easy to decide. If you're the 1 patient in 30,000 who is dead, you're very dead. But would withdrawing the drug cause many more deaths in people who might have been saved by it?

By and large, all that was said in the last "Questions" chapter applies to drugs and medications. When a scientist or a company comes forth with a new drug, or with a new use for an old one, ask: How do you know it works? What is your evidence?

Warning: You aren't likely to find many of the answers in most of the elaborate press kits that accompany the commercial release of many drugs.

Drug trials start in animals. Then clinical (patients) trials are conducted in *phases* – which are hurdles that must be leaped before a drug can win FDA approval.

In a Phase I trial, a new drug is tested in humans for the first time. It has already been studied first *in vitro* ("in glass"), in test tubes (or petri dishes, beakers, or flasks), then *in vivo* ("in something living"), in animals. In Phase I, the investigator tests for human toxicity and for other physiological responses, seeking a dosage range and schedule of acceptable toxicity. Typically, 20 to 80 people (who may be healthy) get the drug in this phase. The doses studied are at first small, then gradually increase.

In Phase II, the drug is tried in more patients (100 to 300) to establish dosages that might be effective. Again, there may be studies of various doses, schedules, and safety margins. Some Phase II studies are, like those in Phase I, open studies, with doctors and patients knowing that a new compound is being tested. Other Phase II studies are randomized and blinded.

78

Phase III means a full-scale clinical trial or trials to pit the drug against other treatments or no treatment. This is the last hurdle before winning FDA approval, and typically involves several hundred to 3,000 patients.

Ideally, Phase III trials should be fully randomized, blinded studies comparing comparable groups of patients. For reasons of necessity or expense, they are sometimes less than perfect. They are sometimes crossover studies (the same patients getting one treatment, then another), and sometimes trials comparing the patients with past medical records (historical controls).

Keep in mind that there are differences in physiological response from patient to patient. There are some spontaneous recoveries, along with the placebo effect, in which some patients respond to anything they are given. All these things make drug testing, at best, something less than a gold-plated assurance that a drug is now "safe" (or really, safe enough to be used) and effective.

But the greatest problem of all is that 1,000 or 3,000 patients are few compared with the many more thousands, or even millions, who may have to get a drug before all its effects and their frequencies become known. And when millions are taking the drug, hundreds or thousands of them will have other complicating medical conditions, or be taking other medications that can affect the value and safety of the new drug. The real safety test of a drug is its use by doctors in general, on patients in general.

It is in this "big but poorly controlled experiment," by one description, that the life-threatening events often turn up. If a drug produces an unwarranted reaction in, say, 1 out of every 25,000 patients, the drug would have to be taken by a quarter million people to produce 10 such reactions. Because of the need to have experience with so many patients, in 2007, the FDA's budget was increased to allow the agency to upgrade its post-market surveillance programs.

Case history: The antibiotic chloramphenicol (Chloromycetin) was approved and given to some 5 million people before the FDA decided that it caused serious blood disorders and death in 1 in perhaps 24,000 to 40,000 patients. The FDA then limited the drug's approved indications to a small number of infections, most commonly typhoid fever, and, when no other drug works, some eye, ear, and skin disorders. Some doctors who said they had never seen an adverse reaction continued using the drug more indiscriminately for years, and reports of deaths kept piling up.

A physician may legally use any licensed drug for any purpose, not just the use approved by the FDA. This is called *off-label* use. However, the FDA does not allow drug firms to promote off-label use. In addition, hundreds of doctors, typically in academic medical centers, are using some unlicensed, experimental drugs on patients under FDA investigational permits.

You can read about licensed prescription drugs, including their noncapitalized generic or scientific names, their capitalized trade names, and their possible side effects and approved uses, in the *Physicians' Desk Reference,* or *PDR* – and about many nonprescription drugs in the *PDR for Non-Prescription Drugs.* But prescription drugs are described in the language approved by the FDA as the labeling or package insert usually seen by pharmacists, not by patients. Unfortunately, the online PDR is available online only to certain professionals.

Reading about all the possible side effects of a drug can be frightening – at times, perhaps unnecessarily so. Dr. Gary Friedman notes that "companies tend to include every possible side effect that has been reported, probably to protect themselves [from lawsuits]."[11] Just the same, a reporter writing about a drug should read the full text.

Animals as Stand-Ins for Us

Animals are the most common research subjects of all. Mice and rats are tested by the millions, other animals by the hundreds or thousands. Scientists use animals for three reasons: to study normal and disease processes in living creatures, to assess the efficacy and toxicity of new drugs, and to test products such as chemicals in the environment and cosmetics for safety.

Animals are often much like people in their reactions, and often very different. The challenge to scientists is to pick the right animal model for the subject – the human disease or risk or physiological change – that is being studied. Armadillos are reasonable models for the study of leprosy, cats for deafness, mice for cancer and epilepsy, rats for diabetes and aging, pigs for heart disease, and dogs for many conditions.

But no animal is a completely satisfactory model for any human disease. Cortisone causes cleft palate in mice, but not in humans. A dose of morphine that can kill a human merely anesthetizes a dog. Arsenic doesn't induce cancer in animals, but does in man.

So it's often said that "mice are not men." Yet in some ways, animals are superior to human beings as research subjects. No experimenter can control all human variables, but a scientist can select an inbred strain of mice with common genetics to make sure that this variability isn't confusing the experiment. *Example*: It's easy to control diet in animals – yet often tough in humans. But watch out: If the animals tested have an identical genetic make-up or are all on the same diet, this does not mimic reality. Except for identical twins, humans vary in their genes and actual human study subjects eat a variety of foods.

Mice and other lab animals also allow experiments to be done that would be too dangerous to do in humans. For example, a "knockout mouse" has one of its genes inactivated (knocked out) – which allows scientists to learn precisely what that particular gene does. Or sometimes a gene will be added to the animal to study its function.

When it comes to determining whether a substance is cancer-causing or has other toxic worries, dosages often must be far higher in animals than in typical human exposures. It takes both large dosages and large numbers of subjects to get an answer in mice, which live only a few years, in a reasonable time at an affordable cost. However, the ability to extrapolate from large doses in animals to much smaller doses in humans is difficult and may not be accurate. Because of this and other shortcomings in using animals for safety testing, toxicologists are now developing new tests using *in vitro*, so-called *critical pathways* that hold the promise of reducing the number of animals needed to determine toxicity.

And animal studies are not without possible biases. Animals, like people, vary from day to day in their physiology and behavior. The position of a cage in a room may affect response; careful researchers rotate cages to avoid this *cage effect*. Animals sometimes have undetected infections.

Although caution is required when extrapolating from animals to man, animals can nonetheless alert us to potential uses for drugs and potential problems of chemicals and other agents. There are many classic animal experiments. In 1945, Howard Florey and Ernst Chain infected mice with streptococci, then injected some of them with the new experimental drug penicillin. All of the untreated mice were dead by the next day; all the treated mice lived.

In extrapolating from animals to man, said a 1984 scientific panel, "the characterization of human risk always requires interdisciplinary evaluation of the entire array of data" – laboratory, animal, and human – "on a case by case basis."[12]

In short, it requires human judgment. And the reporter asking a scientist about an animal experiment should ask much the same questions one would ask about a human experiment.

Were there controls? Were there possible biases? What were the numbers? Is this a good animal species for this test or experiment?

81

Do you think you can extrapolate? What is the biological and medical significance for humans?

Writing About New Tests

Human factors to consider:

Convenience – How easy is it for a patient to take the test? How comfortable? Cancer early-detection experts continue to have trouble getting patients to undergo recommended colon exams. Is there any risk to the patient? And how easy is it for doctors to use the test? Will public and private insurers reimburse the cost of the test?

Speed – How quickly are results available? Speedy results allow treatment to start sooner. *Example*: Some strep-throat tests for children. Also, quick results can identify people who need help before they are lost to follow-up. *Example*: Some HIV tests that can more speedily identify people with this AIDS virus.

Notes

1. Sylvia Pagan Westphal, "Medicare Says It Will Cover Test for Heart Device," *Wall Street Journal*, March 22, 2006.
2. http://www.labresultsforlife.org/news/news_050710.cfm
3. http://www.medscape.com/viewarticle/555533
4. http://abcnews.go.com/print?id=9124113
5. Barbara G. Valanis and Carol S. Perlman, "Home Pregnancy Tests: Prevalence of Use, False-Negative Rates and Compliance with Instructions," *American Journal of Public Health* 72, no. 9 (September 1982): 1034–36.
6. Friedman, *Primer*.
7. American Cancer Society, cancer.org
8. Various news reports, including Shirley Wang, "HPV Vaccine Stirs Economic Debate," *Wall Street Journal*, June 29, 2006. Also, American Cancer Society at cancer.org
9. "False Positive Screening for Cancer Found to be Frequent and Costly," American Association for Cancer Research, December 14, 2004.
10. John Urquhart and Klaus Heilman, *Risk Watch: The Odds of Life* (New York: Facts on File, 1984).
11. Friedman, *Primer*.
12. Interdisciplinary Panel on Carcinogenicity, "Criteria for Evidence of Chemical Carcinogenicity," *Science* 225 (August 17, 1984): 682–87.

7

Vital Statistics

I said to a patient who was an undertaker, "I'm curious. How did you happen to pick me as your physician?" He replied: "Nothing to it. I checked the records and found you wrote the fewest death certificates."

Dr. Philip R. Alper in *Medical Economics*

We can brag about some of our nation's vital statistics. Our nation's death rate is at a record low, and life expectancy is at an all-time high.

Other vital statistics show us where we can improve. The infant mortality rate varies greatly across the country. It ranges from 4.4 infant deaths per thousand live births in Vermont and Maine, to 10.3 in Mississippi and Louisiana, at this writing. And in Sweden it's about 3.[1]

Still other vital statistics may surprise us. The death rate in New York City during the first week of the year 2000 was up 50 percent over the comparable week of 1999. Neither influenza nor any other disease outbreak could explain it.

Experts concluded that many terminally ill people pushed themselves to live longer to see the new millennium arrive – much as, other experts believe, some other people live longer to enjoy a major event such as a family wedding.[2]

Vital statistics track the numbers and trends of births, deaths, diseases, and other life events, such as marriages and divorces. They allow us to

News & Numbers: A Writer's Guide to Statistics, Third Edition. Victor Cohn and Lewis Cope with Deborah Cohn Runkle.
© 2012 Victor Cohn and Lewis Cope. Published 2012 by Blackwell Publishing Ltd.

measure the progress – or lack of it – that our nation, our states, and our cities are making against all sorts of diseases. And they often chronicle the cost and other burdens of illnesses as well.

There are breakdowns, breakdowns, and breakdowns of the figures. We can look at national, state, local, and other data. Vital statistics break down cancer and other diseases by gender, age groups, and in many other ways.

As journalists, we can use these figures to write articles about where we stand, where trends appear to be taking us, and to compare our community's experience with the nation's.

The Numbers of Life and Health

John Graunt, a 17th-century Englishman who was a pioneer in vital statistics, calculated London's three leading causes of deaths in 1632. He called them "chrisomes and infants" (which meant infant deaths, because chrisomes were used as burial robes for babies); "consumption" (tuberculosis and probably cancer and other wasting diseases); and "fever."

In this day of antibiotics and other treatments that have lengthened the average life expectancy, the three leading causes of death in the United States are, in order, heart disease, cancer, and strokes.[3] However, as the population gets older, Dr. Eric Kort and colleagues predict that cancer may soon overtake heart disease worldwide as the leading cause of death, because cancer is often referred to as a disease of aging.[4]

Graunt also developed rates and proportions as ways to describe what he saw, and pointed out how such data might be used to spot problems. "There is much pleasure," he wrote, "in deducing so many abstruse, and unexpected inferences."[5]

Not until the mid–19th century did registration of births and causes of death become at all regular in both the United States and Britain, but Graunt's rates remain central to measuring nature's continuing experiment that is life.

Key rates of death and disease

A rate, to a statistician, is a specific kind of proportion. It tells you "so many per so many" per unit of time – in essence if not those precise words. A rate answers the question: Compared with whom (or what)?

The two most commonly used medical rates – incidence and prevalence – are often confused, even in the medical literature.

An incidence rate is the number of persons who get a disease, divided by the total number at risk (or total given population), per unit of time.

Example: The incidence rate of disease A is 3 percent a year in the United States. That is, in any given year, about 3 percent of all Americans develop this illness.

Incidence measures only new cases or, strictly, new cases that are diagnosed. Often, the true incidence can only be estimated.

A prevalence rate of a disease is the total rate, of both new cases and old cases, in a given population at a given time. It is the total number of persons affected at that time divided by the total population.

If incidence is like an entering class, prevalence is the whole school.

Example: The prevalence rate of condition A in the screening exam at the plant was 1 percent.

(The word "rate" is often assumed in many incidence and prevalence rates.)

Case rate is a term sometimes used to mean a disease's prevalence rate, with *new case rate* referring to the incidence. But be careful – all these terms are often used loosely or carelessly.

Other rates for deaths and illness:

- **A mortality rate** is the incidence of *deaths* per unit of time in a community, nation, or group.
- **A morbidity rate** is the equivalent rate of a *particular disease* or, sometimes, of all illness.
- **Years of potential life lost (YPLL)** is a measure of premature mortality. It ranks causes of deaths by measuring the number of years of life lost, rather than number of lives lost.

For YPLL, experts calculate the years lost from a relatively normal life expectancy of 78 years. For example, a person who dies of heart disease at age 76 counts as only a few years of life lost. A 13-year-old girl who dies in a traffic accident counts as 65 years of life lost. (Note that these statistics are for men and women combined. Actually, the life expectancy for men is a little less than 78 and for women a little more.)

Accidents are the nation's number five cause of death in the United States when calculated in the traditional each-death-counts-as-one way. But accidents rise to number three in YPLL calculations (still behind heart disease and cancer), because many accidental deaths occur at relatively young ages. (Note again: leading causes of death differ slightly for men and women; the figures given here are the combined numbers.)

YPLL is a good way of looking at prevention potential, but it best supplements rather than replaces the regular mortality rate.

Crude rates versus rates that compare

We said that rates answer the question: Compared with what? There are several basic ways of describing populations or groups so that they can be compared:

- **A crude rate,** whether an incidence, mortality, or prevalence rate, simply tells you the number of cases or whatever in a population. It is important to know, but it's no help if you want to know where the disease is concentrated.
- **A group-specific** rate can more tellingly state the number of cases in some subgroup, that is, what proportion of what group is affected.
- **An age-specific rate,** or an age- and gender-specific rate, is often given in 5- or 10-year groupings.
- **A case-fatality rate** is the number of persons dying of a disease divided by the total number who have it. This may be stated per unit of time, or simply as the proportion who eventually die of the condition.
- **The maternal mortality rate** is the number of maternal deaths attributed to childbirth in a year, divided by total live births.
- **An attack rate** is the cumulative count of new cases (in relation to a total population, without specifying a unit of time). But it is commonly used in connection with a specific epidemic or – a term with less emotional charge – outbreak of a disease.
- **An age-adjusted rate** is used when you need to compare two groups that are not comparable in some important way, such as age. For example, one way of arriving at an age-adjusted rate is to choose some standard population – the U.S. population in a particular year, for example – and calculate the number of cases that would occur if the population you are looking at had the same distribution.

Example: The age-adjusted rate for Florida would tell you what Florida's rate would be if that state wasn't a retirement mecca but had a more normal distribution of younger people.

True, you are now dealing with a contrived rate that does not truly describe the population. For that, you may need a crude rate. Yet for many purposes an adjusted rate gives you a clearer picture.

One statistician says, "I think group-specific rates give you the clearest picture of a disease. But say you want to compare two cities. If you just want to know the prevalence of a disease in the two, you should know the crude rates – after all, they tell you how big a problem each city has. But if you want to know why the two cities differ, you must adjust, ideally, by age, gender, race, income, and often occupation. And you'll know even more if you also compare the group-specific rates in the two."

If you did not age-adjust U.S. cancer rates when comparing them from decade to decade, you would not be taking into account that people have been living long enough to get cancer instead of dying from other diseases.

An adjusted rate gives you what statisticians call an *expected rate* compared with the actual observed rate.

Friedman points out that you might want to compare the lung cancer rate in a group of smokers with that in some nonsmokers of various ages. You want to compare the results of smoking, not age, so you age-adjust the nonsmokers' lung cancer rate to the rate you'd expect if they were the same age as the smokers. You can now more accurately see the effect of cigarettes on the smokers.[6]

You'll sometimes see a reference to the *magnitude* of a difference between two groups. That's just its size. Say one group has 100 more cases of a disease than another, or one has a 50 percent greater rate. Those figures are the magnitudes of the difference.

Putting numbers on risks

A difference between two incidence or prevalence rates can be called an *excess rate* or *excess risk* – and an attributable risk if there is a difference in some variable, such as cigarette smoking, that is strongly believed to cause the difference. Investigators like to say that the guilty variable has a "causal role." But that's a phrase you may want to avoid in print, since a typo (or a quick reading) too often changes it to a "casual" role.

You can usefully compare two rates by calculating the ratio of one to the other – that is, dividing one by the other. This gives you the *relative risk*, or *risk ratio*.

Example: If disease A occurs in 50 cases per 100,000 in group X and in 200 per 100,000 in group Y, group Y's risk is four times greater than group X's. This is commonly expressed as a relative risk of 4.

You'll often see a lower number for a relative risk, such as 1.3 or 1.5 – that is, a 30 or 50 percent increased chance of disease, death, exposure, or whatever. A reported relative risk that small may or may not signal a problem, given the limited reliability of observation and other possible variables. Any risk ratio of less than 2.0 may not be meaningful and is a signal for a reporter to ask more questions.

Example of a particularly strong risk ratio: In an American Cancer Society smoking study, the lung cancer mortality rate in nonsmokers aged 55 to 69 was 19 per 100,000 per year; the risk in smokers was 188 per 100,000. Since 188 divided by 19 equals 9.89, the smokers were about 9.9 times more likely to die from lung cancer – their relative risk was 9.9.[7]

A caution when reporting on lung cancer: There are several kinds of lung cancer, some of which are not related to – or "caused by" – either cigarette smoking or second-hand smoke.

Example of a relatively small risk ratio: A disease has a background rate (normal occurrence) of 50 cases per 100,000 people. A study finds 65 cases per 100,000 workers who are occupationally exposed to a certain chemical. This is an increased risk of 30 percent, for a relative risk of 1.3. Other evidence may be needed to show that the chemical is the culprit for this relatively small increase.

To introduce another term: The greater the odds of an association, the greater is the *strength* of the association.

As important as it can be, a risk-ratio figure standing alone doesn't give the full picture. It doesn't tell how many people are at the increased risk – for example, how many people smoke.

And in total lives affected, a large risk ratio for a rare condition may not be as important as a smaller risk ratio for a common illness such as breast cancer.

Two cautions

States are ranked, from best to worst, in everything from infant mortality rates to divorce rates. But often there are only minor differences between some of the states on these lists that would not be considered statistically or practically significant. For example, the 27th-ranked state may be doing almost as well as the 17th-ranked state. These minor differences also can result in large year-to-year changes in your state's position on a list.

The lesson: It's often helpful to report these rankings. It's more helpful, to your readers or viewers, when you point out that your state is close to several other states.

Percentage increases sometimes can be misleading too. A disease outbreak may start with, say, three reported cases. By the time there are 33 cases, there will have been a 1,000 percent increase! By contrast, when 95 percent of a state's youngsters have been immunized against a particular disease, it's impossible to have a large percentage increase. There's no room to go up!

The lesson: When you start with a small base, any significant gain is likely to be large in percentage terms. Use caution so that you don't hype the figures.

Cancer Numbers

The basics:

Numbers that some people call "cure rates" are more properly called "survival rates."

"*Relative* survival rates" tell you what you really want to know about survival.

Different types and *stages* of cancer have different survival rates.

The bottom-line statistics are the cancer death rates and the total number of deaths. The news here is encouraging.

Incidence rates (new cases) can fill out the picture.

Now the details:

Survival rates

What's a cure? Normally, it means no more evidence of disease, no recurrence, and a normal life expectancy – one that would be "expected" without the disease in question. But for cancer, some people sometimes talk of 5-year and occasionally 10-year "cure rates." With many types of cancer, most patients, but not all, who survive 5 years will have no recurrence.

The 10-year rate is sometimes cited too. And it should be, to be honest, for breast cancer and prostate cancer – just two examples of cancers with many deaths after 5 years, or even 10 years later.

In short, the fact that not all cancer patients will survive means that no one can truly tell until years later which patients are cured and which patients are not. Strictly speaking, a cure should mean only that the patient very certainly does not have the disease anymore. Thus, it is more accurate to report 5-year and 10-year "relative survival rates," rather than calling them "cure rates."

Absolute survival (also called *observed survival*) is simply the actual proportion of patients still alive after *X* years, considering deaths from all causes, cancer or otherwise.

Relative survival, the preferred figure, is calculated by adjusting the observed survival to take into account the normal life expectancy of a similar population. In effect, you gauge the effect of cancer alone by using statistical methods to remove the effect of all other causes of death – heart attack, auto accidents, shootings, or whatever.

Where this key rate now stands: The 5-year relative survival rate for U.S. patients with cancer – at all sites in the body combined – is now 65 percent, according to a 2006 report by the American Cancer Society. That's up from about 50 percent in the mid-1970s.[8]

Too many news stories skip mentioning that they are dealing with relative survival. The story may say "65 percent of cancer patients survive." To be honest, we should explain relative survival and use terms such as "survive from cancer" or "survive the effects of cancer." Cancer commonly occurs in older patients, so it's not surprising that many die of other causes.

The increasing push for early detection of some types of cancer is truly helping increase survival. Early detection can find these types of cancers at stages where they are more likely to be treated successfully.

But early detection also can cause a statistical quirk that's called *lead-time bias*. By finding cancer earlier, it starts the "survival-rate clock" running earlier. That can make the apparent length of survival seem longer, when it may not actually be so. *Example:* Say a cancer is detected two years earlier than it otherwise would have been found. For that reason alone, the patient would be expected to survive two years longer from the time of the diagnosis.

Because of this lead-time bias, many experts believe the best way of looking at overall progress against cancer is the death rate.

Deaths, new cases, and other numbers

Death rate and total deaths – The nation's overall *cancer death rate* has been falling, albeit slowly, in the last three decades This rate is the number of cancer deaths per 100,000 Americans. (However, because of the growth of the nation's population, the actual *number of cancer deaths* continued to rise until 2003, when a small decline began.)[9]

New cases – Another important calculation seeks to measure how many new cancer cases are occurring. The *cancer incidence rate* is based on the number of newly diagnosed cases. This rate, for cancer at all sites in the body combined, has been holding relatively steady.

Different types of cancer – There's lung cancer, breast cancer, and many other types. All have one thing in common: uncontrolled growth of abnormal cells, with a threat of spread, or *metastasis*. But survival rates and other statistics can differ markedly from one type to another. The chances of surviving lung cancer, for example, are much lower than surviving breast cancer. And there are different numbers for various subtypes too – for example, different subtypes of lung cancer.

Also, an individual patient's chances of successful treatment are affected by the *staging* of the cancer – whether it has started to spread, or how far it has spread. These statistics can be particularly important for people who have cancer, and for the doctors and nurses who treat them. And they can be important if you are writing about a public figure or anyone else who has cancer.

Still other figures tell you what has been happening in white males, white females, black males, black females, or other groups.

"Cancer Facts and Figures," by the American Cancer Society, has numerous statistical breakdowns. It also has detailed information on how all types of cancer statistics are compiled, as well as general information about cancer. It's at cancer.org.

An important explanation of "cancer sites" terms:

Lung cancer, breast cancer, and all other such terms are based on where the cancer started. Colon cancer, for example, may spread to the liver, but it's still classified as colon cancer because that's where it began in the body.

"All sites" means cancer occurring anywhere in the body, with one major caveat: Some forms of skin cancers that are relatively easy to cure are not counted in some statistics.

Breast cancer's one-in-nine lifetime risk

You may read or hear that a "woman has a one-in-nine risk of developing breast cancer in her lifetime." Some doctors, reporters, and others use such *lifetime risk* numbers to encourage women to have early-detection mammograms – a noble goal. But lifetime risk estimates can be misleading unless accompanied by caveats, which too often are missing.

In "Putting the Risk of Breast Cancer in Perspective" in the *New England Journal of Medicine*, and in a follow-up letter to the editors of that journal, doctors noted: Breast cancer lifetime estimates really mean that an *average* woman has a statistical one-in-nine risk of developing breast cancer *at some point* over the course of her *entire* lifetime. The risk in any single year of life – or even decade of life – is much lower. The older the woman, the greater is that risk.[10] This point needs to be kept in mind when reporting on the risks and benefits of mammography screening for breast cancer. Remember, yearly breast imaging is not aiming to catch one in nine women with breast cancer, because far fewer women than that develop breast cancer in any given year. And mammography is not perfect; it misses some cancers and results in some false positives.

All such estimates are necessarily based on current trends, which could change over time. And some women have higher, some lower, risks than the average, based on the family history of breast cancer and other factors.[11] The doctors urge the news media to avoid scary generalizations. They also might remind women that heart disease is the number one killer of women.

The American Cancer Society now uses age-group breakdowns that can be helpful. The society, in its "Cancer Facts and Figures 2000" report, estimated the risk of an *average* American women being diagnosed with breast cancer:

- at some point before reaching age 40, one in 235;
- at some point between age 40 and 59, one in 25;
- at some point between age 60 and 79, one in 15.

The Cancer Society provides similar calculations for other types of cancer. It's still good to point out that, for an individual, various factors can mean an above-average or a below-average risk. For example, the *average* person's risk of developing small cell lung cancer has little meaning – unless you get a breakdown for smokers and nonsmokers.

Confusing clusters

Small-scale cancer incidence figures are often deceptive. A town or county may report a startling number of cases of some type of cancer in the area of a chemical plant or toxic waste dump. If you investigate, you may find that many U.S. census tracts or municipalities, with no troublesome industrial or other toxic source, have equally large numbers just by chance and the laws of statistical variation.

The same applies to that commonly reported phenomenon the *cancer cluster* – an alarming-sounding concentration of some kind of cancer in a city block or neighborhood. In most cases its cause, if any, remains unresolved. Many – some authorities say almost all – are probably the result of statistical variation, in other words, chance. Only in a few cases is some reasonable possible cause, such as an industrial or environmental hot spot, identified. The same holds true for birth defects, with reports appearing from time to time of an unusual "cluster" in a particular area.

The difficulty for epidemiologists, reporters, and the public alike is distinguishing possible real problem areas from those that only seem to exist. It takes a large number of new "problem cases" to show up against the normal cancer caseload, and it may take 5 to 40 years' exposure for true problem cases to show up (less for some leukemias).

Case history – In the mid-1980s, a spate of news stories reported that cancer had been diagnosed in no less than four New York Giants football players. There was public concern about the chemistry (or atmosphere or something) of the then recently completed New Jersey Meadowlands Sports Complex.

Studies of more than 7,000 people who had worked at the sports complex found that their cancer incidence rate was no higher than the rate in the general population. No dangerous levels of cancer-causing substances were found. And the players' cancers apparently had started before they joined the Giants.

Case closed. From all indications, it was just another coincidence cluster.[12]

Writing about the causes of cancer

A 1984 survey by the federal National Cancer Institute indicated that many people refused to consider healthy changes in lifestyle because they thought that "carcinogens are everywhere in the environment."[13] Public knowledge has since improved – yet maybe not enough. To keep the record straight, lifestyle choices offer by far the biggest opportunities for cancer prevention. The chief things to think about:

Tobacco smoking – which not only causes lung cancer, but plays roles in several other types of malignancies and other diseases – "accounts for some 30 per cent of all cancer deaths," the American Cancer Society notes.

Although for years we were told that simply eating more fruits and vegetables can help reduce the risk of cancer, research results appearing in the *Journal of the National Cancer Institute* in 2010 reported that a study of 478,000 Europeans showed that eating these foods had only a little, if any, effect on preventing cancer. Nevertheless, people are still encouraged to eat lots of fruits and vegetables, because these food groups are associated with a lower risk of cardiovascular disease.[14] However, weight control, and even exercise (both of which affect the body's hormones), can lesson the chances of getting cancer.

Overexposure to the sun is the chief culprit for skin cancer. Yes, there are cancer risks from asbestos, certain chemicals, and other environmental exposure. But when it comes to carcinogens in the air, most people should think first about second-hand tobacco smoke.

For more about all these things, click on the Cancer Society's cancer.org.

Other calculations to consider

You also should know:

- Doctors who treat cancer may report their five-year survival rate even though not all the patients have survived for five years yet. But there's a need to explain why this is.

Example: In 1985, oncologists (cancer doctors) at many centers reported the cumulative results of some newer treatments of breast cancer. Instead of reporting absolute survival alone – how many patients lived exactly how long – they used a *life table method* or *actuarial method*. This allows them to say: Enough of our patients have been followed for five years, and enough for one, two, three, or four years, for us to say with confidence what the five-year survival rate for the whole group will be.

This is considered statistically honest and respectable if completely described. In fact, one statistician says, "It is wrong if it is not reported. It is the only way we can know how we are progressing in this difficult disease." But the method should be described in our news stories too, to be honest.

- A cancer researcher sometimes reports patients' mean or median survival – that is, how long a group of patients have lived on the average by one of these measures. The median does tell you that half of the patients did that well or better. But the measure picked may be the best-sounding one. Neither the mean nor the median tells you how many people have survived how much longer or how briefly. For that, you need to see a fuller explanation or a revealing table or graph.

Shifts, Drifts, and Blips

A death blamed on senility in 1900 would probably have been put down as "general arteriosclerosis" in 1960. Now it probably would be blamed either on cerebrovascular disease (including strokes) or Alzheimer's disease, which is now recognized as a cause of a large proportion of senility and death.

Medical knowledge, medical definitions, doctors' skills, doctors' diagnostic enthusiasms, and the way statisticians code disease all change. Some diseases – such as the connective tissue disorder called lupus – appear to have increased dramatically simply because they are being found more often. Death certificates have been called notoriously inaccurate. The number of autopsies, the most accurate method of identifying cause of death, has dropped sharply in recent years.

These are only a few of the rocks and shoals in determining who died of what and who has what. There are also unexplained or incompletely explained drifts in the statistics, such as the declines in stomach cancer deaths.

The news media also affect disease rates. When reporters write about a particular illness, such as some food-borne malady or Lyme disease, more people may see their doctors with such problems, or the patients may report their illnesses directly to health officials.

Then there was the "Betty Ford blip" in breast cancer incidence. This was a dramatic rise in discovery of new cases for a few years after that First Lady's 1974 breast cancer surgery, along with the publicity that her case generated about breast cancer early detection and surgery.

The same thing happened in 2000, when news anchor Katie Couric had a colonoscopy on national television. Researchers at the University of Michigan Health System and the University of Iowa reported a jump in the number of people showing up at their doctors' offices to undergo this procedure for diagnosing colon cancer early, sometimes in a pre-cancer stage.[15]

Notes

1. Various U.S. government reports; check at cdc.gov and census.gov
2. Robert D. Hershey, Jr., "Rise in Death Rate After New Year Is Tied to Will to See 2000," front-page article in *New York Times*, 15 January 15, 2000.
3. http://www.infoplease.com/ipa/A0005110.html

4. E. J. Kort et al., "Cancer Mortality Rates Experience Steady Decline," *Cancer Research* (August 15, 2009): 69.
5. In Devra Lee Davis, *When Smoke Ran Like Water: Tales of Environmental Deception and the Battle against Pollution*. (New York: Basic Books, 2002).
6. Friedman, *Primer*.
7. Hammond, "Smoking."
8. "Cancer Facts and Figures," American Cancer Society, at cancer.org
9. Denise Gray, "Dip in Cancer Deaths Is Reported, First Decline in U.S. in 70 Years," *New York Times*, February 8, 2006; National Cancer Institute, "Annual Report to the Nation Finds Cancer Death Rates Still on the Decline," 2005–2006.
10. Kelly-Anne Phillips et al., "Putting the Risk of Breast Cancer in Perspective," *New England Journal of Medicine* 340, no. 2 (14 January 1999): 141–44.
11. Barbara B. Harrell, "The One-in-Nine Risk of Breast Cancer," letter to editor, *New England Journal of Medicine* 340, no. 23 (June 10, 1999): 1839–40.
12. Various sources including Joseph Sullivan, "Athletes' Cancers a Coincidence, Study of Meadowlands Site Finds," *New York Times*, July 15, 1989.
13. From various sources, including National Cancer Institute, *Cancer Prevention Awareness Survey*, Technical Report, NIH Publication 84-2677, February 1984.
14. Tara Parker-Pope, "Eating Vegetables Doesn't Stop Cancer," *New York Times*, April 8, 2010.
15. "U-M Study: Katie Couric's Colonoscopy Caused Cross-Country Climb in Colon Cancer Checks," http://www.med.umich.edu/opm/news-page/2003/couric.htm

8

Health Costs, Quality, and Insurance

If I had known I was going to live this long, I would have taken better care of myself.

Casey Stengel, on turning 80

President Obama has signed into law a plan for the most extensive – and some say expensive – health care system overhaul in our nation's history. As its various provisions are phased in, it will guarantee access to health insurance for millions of Americans who have lacked such coverage.[1]

The new law also guarantees continuing controversy.

Critics call it much-too-costly ObamaCare, while supporters see it as too-long-waited-for health care reform. We must watch the numbers to see who's right about what.

Critics charge that the government's costs – including subsidies to help some lower income people buy their insurance – will trigger burdensome tax increases. Watch not only tax measures, but the economic effect on the businesses that pay part of the health insurance costs for their employees. And watch the effect on those businesses that self-insure, that is, pay the health care costs of their employees directly, rather than subsidizing their insurance premiums. (Many officials from both kinds of businesses complain that their costs will go up and their employees' salaries will go down as a result of the new health care law.)

News & Numbers: A Writer's Guide to Statistics, Third Edition. Victor Cohn and Lewis Cope with Deborah Cohn Runkle.
© 2012 Victor Cohn and Lewis Cope. Published 2012 by Blackwell Publishing Ltd.

And watch the economic impact on individuals and families. Supporters of the new law hope that with more widespread health insurance coverage, there will be fewer personal bankruptcies and better health. The numbers will tell us if they're right.

And these supporters see the law as a way to slow the rapid increase in health costs – not stop the increase, but "bend the curve." People with health insurance will be more likely to see a doctor for preventive care, and for earlier treatments of medical problems before these conditions become severe and much more costly to treat, the proponents insist. Watch for evidence of this effect and watch critically for numbers that tell us whether more preventive care and early detection of disease really reduce medical costs. And keep an eye out for cost pressures, as some people with delayed health care needs move into the ranks of insured patients and incur costly medical treatments.

What should you watch for? Use-rates for hospital emergency rooms could be an early indicator of whether improved system efficiency is being achieved. The hope is that with more people having insurance for doctors' office visits, fewer will need to visit emergency rooms, where costs are much higher.

And watch for numbers indicating a shortage of doctors and other health care providers. Already, the country has a shortfall in primary care physicians and in nurses. This is likely to increase with an aging population seeking more medical care. With millions of newly insured people, will the doctor shortage turn into a crisis?

Some critics also fear that with the government so involved, bureaucrats will be tempted to intrude on doctors' decision-making. The government might push for guidelines that would limit coverage for some expensive types of care, these opponents charge. The alarmists predict "death panels." But such problems have already popped up with health insurers, both public (Medicare and Medicaid) and private in recent years. Guidelines can be beneficial – *if* they are based on careful studies with strong numbers showing which treatments work best (see our discussion of Comparative Effectiveness Research in Chapter 2).

The new law also puts tighter controls on health insurance companies, for example, telling them what percentage of premium income must be paid out in benefits, as opposed to salaries or dividends. But, on the other hand, the insurers could benefit from the increase in the number of Americans who buy coverage. Keep your eyes on the dollar numbers. Watch the trends of how much these insurers charge for coverage, their profits and their stock prices, their top executives' pay. And remember, health insurance costs were going up before "ObamaCare."

And again, it will be very important to watch how the new law may affect health outcomes. Will earlier prenatal care lead to a drop in the infant mortality rate? Will death rates from heart attacks and other diseases fall? The numbers will tell us.

Finally, remember that when critics and supporters evaluate the new health care legislation in years to come, they will be looking at more than numbers. Numbers can tell us only so much. For those people who oppose excessive government involvement in the private sector, no statistics are likely to change their minds about the new direction in our country's health care system. And for those whose most important value is seeing more equality in health care insurance coverage, some of the numbers cited above – like increased taxes – won't change their minds.

Separate from the new law, more numbers have become available that can help journalists write about the quality of care offered by individual health insurance plans and hospitals. And many of these numbers are just a few mouse-clicks away. But keep in mind, there isn't any single number that shouts, "Here's the best health plan – or hospital – for everyone!" If anyone claims there is, you probably shouldn't believe it. Health care evaluation isn't that simple.

Instead, most of the numbers show how well a health plan's doctors or a hospital's staff members are doing in specific areas, ranging from making sure that their patients have all appropriate immunizations to caring for heart attack victims with the best available treatment. In some states, hospital death rates also are available, although hospital-to-hospital comparisons can be tricky. Below, we discuss some of the variables that can complicate hospital-to-hospital comparisons.

For all the limits, these numbers are a great starting place for journalists who want to help their readers make more informed and better health care choices. So we'll look first at health plans, then at hospitals, then finally at more things to consider when writing about health costs.

Health Insurance Plans

A good starting point for journalists is www.ncqa.org, the website of the National Committee for Quality Assurance (NCQA). a nonprofit group that accredits health plans and offers various ratings.

Numbers will start tumbling out, telling you how well individual health plans are doing in meeting widely accepted, top-quality-care guidelines for four key chronic illnesses – asthma, diabetes, heart disease, and mental health.

Also check out "Best Health Plans" at the *U.S. News & World Report* website, www.usnews.com, which uses NCQA data in its rankings.

Health officials in your state may have other information about how well various health plans are doing in meeting guidelines for the care of patients with various medical conditions.

Interviewing – Talk to officials of health plans that score both high and low in various measures. If you think it's necessary, ask officials of a high-scoring plan: Are your plan's scores higher simply because your members are younger and, therefore, have easier-to-treat problems or no problems at all? And ask patients what they think. We suggest seeking out those who need and use their health plan the most.

Complaints – Ask your state's insurance commissioner's office, your state health department, and others for any data they may have on complaints about health plans. And any compliments, if they have them too.

Plan-switch rates – Statistics on patients and physicians leaving a health plan, when available, can be analyzed for signs of dissatisfaction. But compare with caution. Patients' switches may be the result of their employers changing plans in the quest for lower rates. And physicians may leave a plan for a variety of reasons.

Writing – Explain to your readers the two key ways that the information can help them. First, some patients who are looking for a particular type of care (for example, heart care) can zero in on those particular numbers to see how well different health plans are doing. Other patients will be most interested in a broader view of how well each plan is doing, because in medicine you never know what your future needs might be.

Caution: Don't make big deals out of very small differences between plans. They may be due more to chance than to medical expertise.

HMO and other terms – In some people's minds, HMOs and managed care plans are synonymous. But managed care is a broader term. It includes Health Maintenance Organizations (HMOs), which require that virtually all care be received through participating doctors and hospitals. And it includes other types of managed care plans (preferred provider plans, etc.) that provide financial incentives for patients to use participating health care providers but still allow some coverage when members use other providers. Keep these differences in mind when comparing health plans.

And now there's a new term, ACOs, which stands for Accountable Care Organizations. This is the name for networks that bring doctors and hospitals into one team. President Obama's new health care law strongly encourages pilot programs to see if these networks will improve efficiency in delivering health care, along with higher-quality care at a lower cost. Mark McClellan, who ran Medicare and Medicaid under President George W. Bush, thinks ACOs are a great idea. But as with every new idea and innovation in health care delivery, there are doubters.[2] So keep an eye out for the verdict on ACOs.

A good contact is America's Health Insurance Plans (AHIP) in Washington, D.C., which represents providers of all types of health coverage. But remember that AHIP represents the industry. Surf the web and find some patient-run or -oriented websites and see what they have to say.

Hospitals

There are two very different types of quality-of-care numbers for hospitals:

1. **Measuring against guidelines** – The federal Medicare program has begun offering these types of numbers for the treatment of heart attacks, heart failure, pneumonia, and surgical infections for most hospitals across the nation.

     The numbers are for the care of adults – not just the senior citizens who are the primary beneficiaries of Medicare. And Medicare's presentation is excellent; check it out at hospitalcompare.hhs.gov.
2. **Looking at outcomes** – Data are available in some states that look at patients' fates, good and bad. These numbers can include improvements, complications, and various other results. But the ones that get the most attention are mortality rates for specific types of care.

Example: A New York state ranking looked at death rates for hospital patients being treated for acute strokes. Twenty-five hospitals came out with high marks; they had proportionally fewer deaths than all of the other hospitals. Other hospitals got middle rankings. But 34 got poor marks for their below-average rankings.[3]

Death rates come with caveats

To seek hospital death-rate data, check with state health departments, employer groups, individual hospitals, and experts who study quality-of-care issues. The numbers may be for all hospitals in a geographical area, or just for *outliers* (hospitals with rates well above or below expected or predicted). But these rates alone still may not tell you which hospitals are the real lifesavers and which may be death traps.

The rates may well have been adjusted for some variables – such as age, gender, previous hospitalization, and the presence of various co-morbidities (illnesses other than the main one causing the admission) – to try to make one hospital's rates comparable with another's. But they may not have been adequately adjusted for the most important variable of all, severity of illness. They also may not have been adjusted for other aspects of patient mix, perhaps including socioeconomic status (poorer may mean sicker) and other characteristics that can affect medical outcomes.

A trauma center, and a hospital that specializes in burns, and a tertiary-care center where other hospitals send their most complicated cases all may have higher death rates than a simpler community hospital.

Experience shows that virtually every hospital official, confronted with a report of high death rates, will say, "Our patients are sicker." And many studies show that there are true differences in care from hospital to hospital.

How can you sort this out? With some good journalistic questioning:

When you are told that a hospital's patients are different, poorer or sicker, or more emergency room cases, and that this explains poorer outcomes, ask:

Can you back that up with statistics, including the numbers about your hospital's population compared with those of other hospitals in the area? Can you point to any hospital with similar patient mixes that has equally unfavorable-sounding rates, in or out of your area?

If you ask about a specific procedure, such as coronary bypass surgery, you may be told that a hospital's high mortality does not mean it isn't giving superior care. Ask:

Is this hospital doing enough of these procedures to be one of the most experienced and successful hospitals? Or is it treating so few patients of this kind that its physicians and staff can't possibly get enough experience to be among the most skilled?

Dr. Sidney Wolfe, director of the Health Research Group founded by Ralph Nader, discussed a federal health agency's release of a small number of hospital mortality rates in 1986:

Of 33 hospitals with an elevated coronary bypass mortality rate, 24 were doing fewer than 100 operations a year. The lowest mortality rate among them was 14 percent. "That's just unconscionable," Wolfe said.

Conversely, the hospitals with lower-than-expected mortality rates, all under 2 percent (a rate seven times lower), did more than 300 bypass operations each year on Medicare patients alone. "What this tells us is that hospitals that are doing very few of these operations, or any others, shouldn't be doing them at all," Wolfe concluded.

Researchers came up with a broader estimate in the March 2000 issue of the *Journal of the American Medical Association*. About 4,000 lives a year might be saved nationwide if surgical patients used only hospitals that had high volumes for selective types of surgery, based on other statistical studies linking volume to mortality rates. But more study is needed to confirm all such estimates, both the research report (which focused on California surgical patterns) and an accompanying editorial (which took the national perspective) cautioned.[4]

If you are still troubled about a hospital's mortality rate, ask yourself, ask doctors, ask others: Would you go to this hospital, or send someone in your family there?

And ask hospital officials: Has your hospital made any changes to improve care, or will it at least be considering changes? This could include changes in medical staff privileges (who can do what kind of surgery), among other things.

Even when a hospital has a relatively low mortality rate, ask: Do you have any special programs that may have helped? But if the hospital primarily attracts an economically upscale, relatively healthy population, ask about that too.

Writing the story – Medicare's website that compares hospitals provides excellent information that can help you explain things to your readers or viewers. Again check out the *U.S. News & World Report* website, usnews.com, to see how they do their hospital rankings.

Hospital errors

A 1999 (updated in 2007) study by the Institute of Medicine (IOM), an arm of the National Academies (formerly the National Academy of Sciences), analyzed various studies that had looked at medical errors, particularly in hospitals, and found cause for grave concern. The IOM concluded that such accidents caused the deaths of 44,000 to 98,000

Americans in hospitals each year due to avoidable errors. The report, while controversial, has stirred hospitals to do better.[5]

Serious hospital errors most often occur in busy settings such as intensive care units (ICUs) and emergency rooms. But there are other problems as well. One major concern has been medication mix-ups and overdoses. Some may be caused when drugs have confusingly similar names – or by some doctors' poor handwriting. Computerized systems may help.

Another helpful tool in reducing hospital errors may be checklists, similar to the ones people take with them to the grocery store. The *New England Journal of Medicine* reported on a study that tested a checklist of best practice procedures. The result? After implementation of the checklist, complications – including infections at the site of surgery and the need for unplanned reoperations – fell dramatically.[6] And at Johns Hopkins University and Hartford Hospital in Connecticut, new safety programs in the ICU resulted in decreases in medication mistakes, mortality rates, lengths of stay, and the number of days patients are on a ventilator.[7]

No one is saying that all errors could be eliminated in hospitals, where many emergency decisions have to be made in rapid-fire order. And even very small mistakes may be life-threatening for a seriously ill, hospitalized patient.

"To err is human, but errors can be prevented," the Institute of Medicine's report said. Or at least errors can be reduced. And hospitals are making major efforts to do just that.

State figures on serious hospital errors are available from some state health departments. Also check with experts studying the issue, and with patient-advocacy groups.

Numbers to watch – How many such errors are being reported? Is there a clear downward trend? Which hospitals have the most reported errors? And are those hospitals simply doing a better job of studying and acknowledging such cases?

Health Care Costs

Medical costs turn some of the normal rules of economics topsy-turvy.

It's the customers who decide whether to buy a new or used car. It's the customers who decide which groceries to buy at what price. But doctors, health insurers, and hospitals – rather than the customers (patients) – make most of the key decisions that affect how much is spent on medical care. The doctors typically decide what tests a patient gets, what drugs to buy, whether a patient goes to a hospital, whether surgery is done, and when the patient should return for more medical care. And doctors feel the constant tugs of insurers' guidelines and hospitals' policies when making their decisions. Sick patients aren't thinking about bargains, they just expect the very best of care.

And in many cases, it's not the direct costs that consumers feel or *even know*. It's the ever-spiraling costs of their health plan or other insurance coverage.

You may be told that, to promote competition, there's a need to build a new hospital, or start some expensive new program. Or you may be told that some new approach to health insurance will spur that competition. If a new restaurant opens up across the street from another restaurant, price competition might result. But hospitals aren't like restaurants and a new hospital in town doesn't necessarily mean that competitive pressure will cause costs to go down. And you might be told that something entirely new will control health costs. Maybe. But because of the complexity of the system, consider all cost-control claims with a prove-it-to-me spirit.

Dollars watch

Here are the some basics to keep in mind when writing about key aspects of health care costs:

1. **Any treatment** – When you write about a surgical or other treatment, consider all the costs. That includes: Hospital as well as doctor costs. Drugs for however long they'll be needed – maybe for days, sometimes for a lifetime. And any other costs such as implants when used, rehab when needed, and so on.
2. **Who pays?** – If there is any doubt, ask whether a treatment is covered by health insurance. That can be the biggest factor of all as far your reader or viewer – the patient – is concerned.
3. **Caution about health plan trends** – From time to time, big business firms will report the "good news": The increases in their spending for employee health insurance have finally begun to slow. But wait! In most such cases, it turns out that the companies are just having their employees pick up more of the costs.

Ask: What's happening with the total premium cost – the employer and employee shares combined?

4. **"Big picture" cost trends** – Price increases are only part of the story. There's more total health care spending because of the growth and aging of the population. There's also more spending to treat new diseases, and to treat old diseases better. Consider all as you write about health care cost trends. A good way of viewing the big picture nationally:

About 15 percent of the nation's Gross Domestic Product (the total of all goods and services produced) now goes for all aspects of health care. This means roughly one out of every seven dollars in our economy. This is up from 7 percent in 1970.[8]

Preventive medicine efforts – ranging from immunizations to weight control – clearly offer important benefits. But if you have any lingering doubts that the medical cost picture is complex, consider the ...

The stop-smoking paradox

Conventional wisdom long assumed that cigarette smoking costs society millions or billions of dollars, by increasing the risk of heart disease, cancer, and other expensive-to-treat illnesses. A 1997 study by Dutch researchers, reported in the *New England Journal of Medicine,* concluded otherwise.

Smoking may actually save society money in the long run, because smokers don't live as long as other folks. They often die of smoking-related diseases before reaching the age where chronic illnesses give a huge push to health costs.

But don't jump to the conclusion that the Dutch researchers think smokers should continue to puff away. Far from it.

"We believe that in formulating public health policy, whether or not smokers impose a net financial burden ought to be of very limited importance," they said. The important thing is that smoking takes an unacceptable heavy toll in death, disease, and their effects on families. "The objective of a policy on smoking should be simple and clear: Smoking should be discouraged."[9]

From time to time, studies raise questions about the costs of various other prevention strategies. But if they save lives or prevent disability, there's great human value in that.[10]

Notes

1. The information on hospital death rates is based in part on an April 1987 health executive training program sponsored by the American Medical Review Research Center and on a paper and sample questions a coauthor of this book (Cohn) prepared. Among speakers whose knowledge we drew on were Andrew Webber, American Medical Peer Review Organization; and Drs. Robert Brook, University of California at Los Angeles and Rand Corporation; John Bunker, Stanford Medical Center; Mark Chassin, Rand Corporation; Carlos Enriquez, Peer Review Organization of New Jersey; Sanford Feldman and William Moncrief, Jr., California Medical Review, Inc.; Harold Luft, University of California at San Francisco; Marilyn Moon, American Association of Retired Persons; Helen Smits, University of Connecticut; and Sidney Wolfe, Public Citizen Health Research Group. The health-plans information is based in part on extensive interviews by Victor Cohn. A detailed look at the subject is in the booklet: *A Newsperson's Guide to Reporting Health Plan Performance*, prepared by Cohn and distributed by the American Association of Health Plans.
2. Alec MacGillis, "For Health-Care Networks, Is Bigger Always Better?" *Washington Post*, August 16, 2010.
3. Milt Freudenheim, "Report Assays Death Rates at Hospitals," *New York Times*, November 25, 2002.
4. Adams Dudley, "Selective Referral to High-Volume Hospitals," and an accompanying editorial, *Journal of the American Medical Association* 283, no. 9 (March 1, 2000): 1159–1166 and 1191–93.
5. http://www/nap.edu/catalog.php?record_id=9728 and http://www.nap.edu/catalog.php?record_id=11623
6. Peter Pronovost et al. "An Intervention to Decrease Catheter-Related Bloodstream Infections in the ICU," *The New England Journal of Medicine* (December 28, 2006): 355.
7. John Kasprak and Saul Spigel, "Hospital ICU Checklist, December 19, 2007. http://www.cga.ct.gov/2007/rpt/2007-R-0728.htm
8. Marc Kaufman and Rob Stein, "Record Share of Economy Is Spent on Health Care," *Washington Post*, January 10, 2006, and other news reports.
9. Jan J. Barendregt et al., "The Health Care Cost of Smoking," *New England Journal of Medicine* 337, no. 15 (October 9, 1997): 1052-57. Also, a news report on the journal article by John Schwartz, "Health Savings for Nonsmokers Disputed," *Washington Post*, October 9, 1997.
10. Spencer Rich, "A Costly Ounce of Prevention," *Washington Post*, August 29, 1993. Also, Laurie Jones, "Does Prevention Save Money?" *American Medical News*, January 9, 1995.

9

Our Environment

When you come to a fork in the road, take it.

Yogi Berra

The gushing blowout of the Deepwater Horizon oil well in the Gulf of Mexico shows how gigantic an environmental disaster can be. Meanwhile, smaller yet important environmental stories are unfolding all the time, posing their own journalistic challenges.

A community, puzzled over some strange illnesses, discovers that it is sitting on a toxic dump. Rivers and the air that we breathe become polluted, sometimes severely so. Men and women become ill after exposures to chemicals in their workplaces. Parents are shocked to learn that some toys they've bought for their kids are contaminated with toxic substances.

Many of these events do not injure large numbers of people, as far as we can tell. Yet thousands upon thousands of people are scared or concerned. We have been told too often that something is safe, only to learn later that this assurance was wrong or that new data change the picture.

Peering into the future, there are bigger worries. What might go wrong at a nuclear power plant? How might global warming affect our planet – and our community?

There are TV news specials and big headlines about all of this. The news media may be accused of overstating, needlessly alarming, emphasizing the worst possible case, reporting unsupported conclusions – or

News & Numbers: A Writer's Guide to Statistics, Third Edition. Victor Cohn and Lewis Cope with Deborah Cohn Runkle.
© 2012 Victor Cohn and Lewis Cope. Published 2012 by Blackwell Publishing Ltd.

being falsely reassuring. Stung by the criticism, we reporters may write "on the one hand, on the other hand" stories, which don't help our readers or viewers figure out if one hand is holding the most credible evidence. What's a reporter to do?[1]

This chapter will look at the three major national environmental policy issues: The Gulf oil spill, global warming and nuclear power. But first, here's a more general look at questions to raise when environmental issues develop:

Let the Questions Fly

Two starter questions that you can ask when someone tells you that there's an environmental problem: What are your specific claims? What's your evidence? As you probe further, ask all the questions that you need to determine:

1. **What is the specific risk, and is it great or small?** What numbers are available?
2. **Under what circumstances?** Is the risk already reaching people? Or will a toxic chemical have to slowly seep into the water supply for the public health to be endangered? Or must something else happen? How might all this unfold?
3. **How certain – or uncertain – is this?** If the evidence is strong, tell your readers or viewers the specifics. If the studies are weak or conflicting, say so. If no one knows, say so. Needed qualifiers add credibility to a report.
4. **What can be done to reduce any risk?** This may include personal actions, or a new law or regulations, or better enforcement of existing regulations, or changes in business or farm practices, or some other actions. Or a combination.
5. **What are the alternatives?** Are there any benefits from what's posing the risk? Who benefits? How do they benefit? How do you weigh the benefits versus the risks? We do need electrical power and waste disposal sites – but there are questions about size, how to do it, and where.

We need to raise questions on both sides of any environmental issues.

For starters, we should be suspicious of sweeping claims such as "substance A causes everything from ingrown toenails to cancer." Substances can have multiple effects, but broad statements are very suspicious until proven otherwise. It's more likely that substance A causes disease B or increases the risk of disease B – although that too must be supported by evidence.

And when cancer is involved, there are special considerations: What kinds of pollutants or other exposure are we talking about? What kinds of cancer? What's known about the cause of this type of cancer? Are there enough cases to be distinguished from other cancers occurring for other reasons? Careful study is always needed.

Then there are specific questions to ask officials and others who play down or deny a risk. The following are based primarily on a checklist prepared by Dr. Peter Montague at Princeton University:[2]

- **When you are told about "safe averages,"** remember that we often encounter hazards as individuals or small groups. If an industrial plant releases a toxic substance, the most important thing is not the average amount that gets in the air, but the amount downwind of the plant where people will breathe it. Ask: What does this mean to individuals? Are children, pregnant women, asthmatics, or any other group particularly vulnerable? What does this mean to your community?
- **When you are told there is "no immediate threat,"** ask: Is there a delayed risk? Cancer and some other problems may develop many years later.
- **When you are told "there is no evidence of hazard,"** ask: Has a scientific study been done?
- **When you are told a hazard is "negligible"** or "nonhazardous," ask: What are the numbers? What would you do? Would you eat or drink it? Would you raise your children in its presence? What do you think the public should do?
- **And when looking further at a risk–benefit or cost–benefit analysis,** ask: Who bears the risk? Who pays the costs? Who gets the benefit? Have those at risk given their informed consent?

Environmental risks aren't limited to threats to human health or animals' wellbeing. We all enjoy clean air and water, so that alone is an excellent reason to keep them clean. But our writings should make clear what types of risks and concerns we are talking about. The emphasis in this chapter is on risks to humans, although the need for sound data applies to the other areas as well.

Checking the Numbers

To influence us, someone may cite an annual death toll, or deaths per thousand or million people, or per thousand persons exposed. Or we may be given deaths per ton of some substance, or per ton released into the air, or per facility. And then there are the nuclear power industry's "deaths per reactor year" calculations.

If you think a different figure is more appropriate, ask for it. Or ask the other side in a controversy what figure it thinks is most appropriate. And you can ask people on both side of a controversy: "Have I been asking the right questions?"

Many points in earlier chapters apply to environmental reporting. Some key ones: Look for statistical significance in the numbers. Give added weight to a study when its findings are in line with earlier research on the subject. And remember the healthy-worker effect, which is so important in environmental reporting that it bears repeating:

You look at the workers exposed to substance A, find that they are actually healthier than the general population, and exonerate the substance – possibly wrongly. Workers tend to be healthier and to live longer than the population in general; they have to be relatively healthy to get their jobs and then to keep working. More research is needed; the numbers must be carefully analyzed.

But when there is a clear problem, don't jump to the conclusion that some suspect chemical in the workplace is the culprit. It might be an above-average rate of cigarette smoking by the workers, or something else. More research and more numbers are called for in all such situations.

Complexity and Assessments

Someone may hear of a nearby environmental threat and say, "That's why I've been sick!" It's a human enough reaction, sometimes right, often wrong. On the other hand, some long-term danger may lurk, yet people remain unaware of it because it's not yet causing problems.

In some situations, people may be affected by interactions between two or more chemicals or substances, making risk analysis particularly tricky. Or there may be no reason for concern, but safety can be hard to pin down too.

Humans can't be treated like lab rats in the quest to find the answers. It would be unethical to expose people, in a controlled experiment, to a chemical expected to cause cancer or some other serious problem.

Animal and lab research, historical data, and studies of exposed people with a comparison group often help sort things out. Yet sometimes we are left with more uncertainty than we would prefer. Decisions still may be needed.

And even when there are risks, there may be costs and practical concerns as well. In some such cases, part of the consideration may be a *risk assessment.* This is often a necessary way of using studies, facts, and conjectures to make a practical assessment of risk, whether the risk of PCBs (polychlorinated biphenyls) or of not installing air bags in our cars.

Risk assessment often gets stepped up to *risk–benefit assessment,* weighing both the probable bad and the probable good. In deciding on the location for a waste disposal plant, how do we weigh the concerns of the small number of people who may live near the site with the much larger number of people whose wastes will fill the site?

Other things make this even trickier. How do you put a cost on a human life or even on a pretty hilltop view? The risk–benefit process involves not only science, but psychology, culture, ideology, economics, values, and politics.

Nevertheless, risk–benefit assessment can get all facts and uncertainties out on the table for public consideration. Despite the potential problems, you can tell your readers what's known and what's unknown about environmental risks, controversies, and studies.

Key Issues: Climate, Nuclear Plants

Here are checklists for reporting climate change and nuclear power:

Global warming – There's now a scientific consensus that human activities are playing key roles in the Earth's rising surface temperatures. Smokestacks and tailpipes emit carbon dioxide and other "greenhouse" gases, which let sunlight in but tend to keep heat from radiating back into space.

What's ahead: The experts believe that the Earth's warming will continue to accelerate – unless something is done to reduce emissions of the heat-trapping gases. But climate trends are complex. There's still spirited debate on how much and how quickly the temperatures will rise. And there are some scientists who do not think that human activity is contributing to climate change, but they're a minority.

Potential consequences: Global warming could discombobulate weather patterns. It could bring flooding in coastal areas as ice caps melt. It could affect disease rates (causing more heatstroke, insect-borne threats, etc.), disrupt agricultural patterns, and trigger other havoc.

Complicated mathematics: Because temperature records around the world were not recorded until relatively recently in history, scientists need to gather indirect data in order to determine whether today's temperatures are indeed warmer than they've been in the past. So scientists from a variety of disciplines take measurements of such things as tree rings and the thickness of Arctic ice to discern ancient patterns. And in order to predict the future, scientists rely on *computer modeling*.

Computer modeling uses software to create mathematical models that simulate the behavior of a variety of systems under differing conditions. For example, economists model how the economy will perform if taxes are raised or lowered. In the case of climate, scientists want to know what will happen to the world's temperatures if we continue our current use of carbon-emitting sources of energy. What if we lower our carbon output by 10 percent? By 20 percent? And what will happen to the spread of bacteria-borne diseases if the Earth continues to warm up? Although computer modeling has become impressively sophisticated, remember the rule of GIGO (garbarge in, garbage out) and read more about that in Chapter 12. So ask the scientists you interview what assumptions and data are going into the computer. Before reporting on results that depend on computer modeling, we recommend that you read "A Skeptic's Guide to Computer Models" by John Sterman of the Sloan School of Management at MIT.[3]

Key questions: Is strong action needed now – or can big decisions wait? Skeptics favor the mildest estimates, but: What if the worst-case predictions are right?

Numbers to watch: Greenhouse gases emissions. Temperature changes over time. Polar ice melting.

Nuclear power[4] – Proponents of nuclear power are urging the building of new plants. They point out that nuclear plants don't pollute the air with fossil-fuel emissions, and say they are needed and safe. Critics cite Three Mile Island, an accident that ruined the power plant, although there were no adverse health risks to the public or workers.

Key questions: How safe – or risky? What about disposal of old but still radioactive fuel? Are plants a tempting target for terrorists?

Numbers to watch: How much growth in electrical power is needed? How many new nuclear power plants will the industry propose? How many (if any) get built? How much "spent fuel" is building up, awaiting permanent disposal?

Six Case Studies: Minds, to Gulf Oil

Mind tricks – In some cases, people can even worry themselves sick. In Washington, D.C., some barrels that were mislabeled "Hazard – Radioactive" rolled off a truck. Even though there was no radiation, the workers cleaning up the mess fell ill. Such weird cases are a reminder that, at times, the power of suggestion can be very powerful indeed. Yet until proven otherwise, illnesses must be taken seriously.

Synergy – The synergistic effect occurs when two substances work together to create unexpectedly large effects: The combined risk is greater than the sum of the substances' risks acting by themselves. Some types of environmental exposures are concerns. One example cited by the federal National Cancer Institute on its website:

Cigarette smokers, on average, are 10 times more likely to develop lung cancer than nonsmokers. For nonsmokers who work with asbestos, the risk is about five times greater than for people in the general population: "By contrast, smokers who are heavily exposed to asbestos are as much as 90 times more likely to develop lung cancer than are non-exposed individuals who do not smoke."

Limits of science – It's useless to ask, "Can you guarantee that X doesn't cause male pattern baldness?" Science can't prove a negative like that.

As one statistician explains, probability "practically guarantees that a small number of studies will show some 'statistically significant' findings if enough studies are carried out. As a result, we can never be 100 percent sure that ... no-association ... is true."[5]

Yet when study after study agrees on anything, the uncertainty can become vanishingly tiny. So from a practical standpoint, science does amazingly well in telling us what we should worry about, and what's not worth worrying about.

Sometimes there's just enough doubt to cloud an issue. Take the long-simmering concern that cell phones might cause brain tumors. Then two major studies in 2000 appeared to acquit the cell phones. Typical of careful comment by experts, these two studies are "the best information to date, and they provide much reassurance."[6] Yet further research has found just enough vague hints that ill-effects *might* occur to keep the controversy alive. More research is coming. But check to see who sponsored the research. Was it the cell phone companies?

What's a journalist to do on all such issues? You can cite the lack of evidence – or the weakness of evidence – that a problem exists. You can be even more reassuring when you can point to multiple studies that have looked for evidence of a risk and come up short. But avoid using the word "proof" in discussing safety, and be suspicious of those who do.

The next two case studies involve interesting environmental history, whose points still prevail:

Two-handed numbers – During a 1990 debate over provisions in the Clean Air Act, a law was proposed to remove more auto-tailpipe emissions. The old law called for a 96 percent reduction in emissions. The new law would have increased the 96 percent to 98 percent.

The auto industry called it an expensive and meaningless two percentage point increase in removal. Environmentalists said that it would result in a 50 percent decrease in the remaining automobile pollution.[7]

Both viewpoints pass math muster, demonstrating that how you word something can make it sound trivial or important, so in cases like this, we suggest reporting both. And that could provide a good lead-in to specifics about what it all means to your readers or viewers.

Expertise as an issue – In some cases, experts may be part of the problem, noted Baruch Fischhoff, professor of engineering and public policy at Carnegie Mellon University in Pittsburgh.[8] Two of his examples:

"The chemists and entomologists [insect experts] who formulated DDT knew and thought little about the fragility of birds' eggs, which was another profession's department." The Three Mile Island nuclear power plant accident in Pennsylvania in 1979 was due, in part, to engineers who designed that plant's system "making unrealistic assumptions about how hard it would be" to operate it.

The bottom line here: Reporters may need to talk not only to experts on both sides of an issue, but to other experts in diverse fields.

That leads to a more recent example of how journalists' use of expertise played out well:

Deepwater Horizon – The gigantic oil spill that gushed from the wrecked well in the Gulf of Mexico spread through one of the nation's most important commercial fishing areas, then onto beaches and other vulnerable shores. And journalists quickly spread out to find the oceanographers, biologists, chemists, physicians, economists, and others who could shine scientific light on the human, wildlife and other impacts.

Many different types of numbers – from measurements of the oil flow, to the counts of people and wildlife affected, to dollar figures – have played major roles in telling this story. And as we noted in the first chapter, the early coverage of this saga played a key role in kicking government action into high gear.

A Questions Bank

This section offers a depository of more questions that you can draw on as needed.

Questions about the scientists

Some scientists have strongly felt political, social, or economic affiliations, and they might not reveal them to you unless you ask. This does not mean that their work or assertions should not be judged on their own merits. Almost everyone is connected to something and has opinions and biases.

Still, you can ask: What are your personal values on this subject? Have you taken public stands on this issue? Do you belong to any organization that has taken similar positions? What government agencies, or companies, or other groups have supported your research?

If questioning a member of a political administration who is stating some conclusion or policy, ask or find out: What is the administration's policy on this? Is your conclusion the same? Have people outside the government come to the same conclusion?

Opinions, affiliations, and sources of financing are normally not indictments. The public still has a right to know them.

Some scientists on all sides – industry, government, environmental groups – "make sweeping judgments on the basis of incomplete, and hence inadequate, data," emphasize their own views, and suppress or minimize conflicting evidence, a Twentieth Century Fund task force concluded.[9]

Yet keep in mind these words from Dr. Gary Friedman: "Ultimately we must all rely on the integrity and objectivity of the researcher, and the basic scientific process of repetition of studies by other investigators."[10]

Questions for evaluating hazards

Dr. Peter Montague and others offer specific suggestions and questions to help evaluate environmental and chemical hazards. (The language in this section is in largest part, but not entirely, Montague's.)

Is this material toxic? How does it get into the environment? Is it vented into the air, discharged into sewage systems, disposed of as wastes?

Is it soluble in water? If so, it tends to be mobile – the world is a wet place. What water supplies could this contamination reach? What towns take their water from this water supply? What's the effect on drinking water?

Is it soluble in lipids – fatty tissue – like DDT is? This makes our bodies repositories.

Will it enter food chains and concentrate? We're at the top of many chains.

Is it likely to become airborne as a gas or dust? Will it then go into the lungs and pass into the bloodstream?

Will it break down – biodegrade – in the environment, or stay around a long time? How long? Are any of its breakdown products also toxic?

What are the substance's hazards to the environment other than the human health impact? Can it migrate to groundwater and cause a bad taste? Can it kill fish, birds, insects, or plants (other than its target species, if a pesticide or herbicide)? What studies have been done to gauge this?

You can ask officials and experts: Would you eat or drink substance A? What are you doing about it? What do you think the public should do?

If a genetically modified organism (GMO) is being introduced into the environment, ask: What effect will this have on the natural plants and animals in the region? What studies have been conducted to test the safety of the new plant or animal?

To those who say, "We don't know the answers," ask: Are you going to try to find out? Is a study planned, by you or by others?

Here are some tips to help judge the size of a hazard – when the numbers needed for such comparisons exist:

How does it compare with background levels? This is important to do whenever possible. Background radiation and natural toxins in food may have some effect on humans, but they are usually the least hazardous we can expect.

A rule of thumb (not always true, but a good guideline to decide whether something deserves serious investigation): A 10 percent increase above natural background levels is something to pay attention to. A factor-of-two increase (a doubling) should be of real concern, unless the original risk was miniscule. A factor-of-10 increase is big; a factor-of-100 increase, very big.

How does it compare with standards for workers? If there is no natural background level, see if there are federal or state standards for workers. It is common to assume that the general public will be adequately protected by a contamination level 10 to 100 times lower than that permitted in the workplace.

The public also, of course, includes infants, the elderly, the chronically ill, urbanites who breathe a mixture of many contaminants, and many people who are more sensitive than others. Thus the reasoning that the public will be protected by a standard 10 to 100 times tighter than a workplace standard has its limits, but it is probably sound as a general rule in the absence of information to the contrary.

Are there drinking water standards or air standards that apply? If state and federal standards exist but are in conflict, give both. The public debate will be heated up, all to the good.

PPB Alert: A company was dumping only 10 gallons of a chemical onto the ground a year – "really no problem," the company said, though it reached the groundwater. Yet if this chemical poses a problem at concentrations measured in a few parts per billion (ppb), there might be a problem. More questions are in order.

What if no standards exist, which is often the case? You can only ask a series of fundamental questions of experts (or reference books) and try to put together a best guess.

When considering an individual's dose of something in the water or air: It's useful to know that a human's daily fluid intake averages two quarts, and the average human breathes 23 cubic meters of air daily.

If you can learn or determine a lethal dose (LD) or toxic dose, divide it into the total amount of the substance involved to determine the total number of doses that you're dealing with.

Who's responsible? When there is an accident or an environmental or other chemical problem, ask: Who has the legal responsibility for compensation, for a clean-up, for a solution? What is going to be done immediately – or as soon as possible – to decontaminate or try to control this problem? How is exposure – in the workplace, in the general environment – to be controlled in the future? Keep in mind that quick fixes aren't always the best fixes.

When someone says, "This solution will be state-of-the-art, the very best technology can do," that may be true. But ask: Is this an adequate solution – for public health and safety and for protection of the environment? Remember how many "solutions" were attempted to fix the Deepwater Horizon oil spill before the right one was found.

Is the solution workable? Have the management and operation been well thought out? Has human error been anticipated? Will there be continuous monitoring for some unexpected release?

What will happen if someone makes a serious error? To quote columnist Ellen Goodman, "We are stuck here in the high-tech, high-risk world with our own low-tech species."

Group versus individual risk – Someone says don't worry, a toxic waste disposal site is being built in a rural area where few people live.

True, fewer people will be affected if a chemical brew leaks from the site. But for an individual who lives near the site, regardless of where the site is, the risk remains the same.

We add these possible questions – from various experts – for two specific types of hazards:

Pesticides – Has a federal tolerance, or maximum permitted residue, been set for this product? What foods does it cover? What information was used to set the tolerance? Has use increased since the tolerance was set? Is the tolerance still adequate? Are there recent studies of actual residue in food?

Radiation – In reporting on radiation (whether it's on the Three Mile Island scale or something smaller but still worrisome), distinguish between the radiation that has actually reached people and any radioactive fallout in the air, water, soil, crops, and milk. Ask:

- *What are the fallout levels* in the air, water, and soil? How much has reached or may reach food supplies?
- *What chemical elements* are involved? (Radioactive iodine, plutonium, etc., may enter and affect the body in different ways.)
- *What is the current or expected whole-body exposure?* How much is a lethal dose – one causing imminent death? How much is a harmful dose? From the standpoint of cancer? Of future birth defects? Of early death?
- *How do the radiation levels compare* with the area's natural background – the radioactivity always present in air, water, soil, and rocks? A comparison with background levels may sometimes reveal almost no added increment. But be aware that, in one environmentalist's words, "this is a time-honored way to minimize adverse effects."

Questions for Evaluating Studies

The general advice in previous chapters applies to environmental studies as well as other claims. But some environmentally tailored questions may help. Pick and choose those that you need to ask a researcher, official, or someone else:

The basics – What is your evidence? What do you base your conclusions on? What type of study have you done (or what study are you citing in support of your views)? Have other experts reviewed it?

The numbers – When you are told about rates and excess risks: What are the actual figures? How many people are affected out of how large a population? What sort of rate would you expect normally? What are the rates elsewhere?

Are your assumptions based on human or animal data?

If human data – How many people have you looked at? Are your study groups large enough to give you confidence that your conclusions are correct?

Sampling – Do you believe that your sample (the people studied) is representative of the general population? Or of the population you're trying to apply it to? How did you pick your sample? At random?

Keep in mind that volunteers may be people with a gripe.

Example: A questionnaire, sent to a large group of women, asked them if they had received breast implants and how their health was. Only a fraction of the women returned the questionnaire. But among those who did, a surprisingly large number had breast implants. And they reported a large number of health problems. Some experts took the survey's results to mean that the implants were very unsafe. Other experts countered that women who had a gripe about their implants were more likely to have taken the time to return the questionnaire. Other studies have done a better job of sorting out which problems probably are, and which problems probably aren't, caused by breast implants. But the debate continues.

Cases – If conclusions are based on cases – people supposedly affected by some agent: Have you yourself observed the effects in the people you're talking about, or did you have to depend on their recall?

To gauge toxicity – Was everyone who was exposed affected? Usually this is not the case; when it is, it may indicate an unusually high level of toxicity. Do you have any information on the people's exposure?

If the reported illnesses are serious: Did you examine the people reportedly affected? Who made what diagnoses? Were the diagnoses firm? Do you have any information on their exposures?

Limits and doubts – How certain are you? What is really known and what is still unknown? What is the degree of uncertainty? Are you missing any data that you would like to have?

Could the association or result have occurred just by chance? What are your figures for statistical significance? Check the P value or confidence level. (See the discussion on probability in Chapter 3.)

Are you concluding that there is a cause-and-effect relationship? Or only a possible suspicious association?

What possible weaknesses or qualifications still apply to your findings or conclusions? Could something else – any other variables, any biases, anything else – have accounted for your results? You should look favorably on a researcher's clear, forthright statement on such matters, unless the defects are overwhelming.

Exposures and dosages – Have you found a dose–response relationship? How much of this substance causes how much harm? Or is the answer "We don't know"? Are you assuming that there is an effect at a low dose because you believe there is a no-threshold dose below which exposure is not dangerous? Do we know the relationship between low and high doses? Or is there some other reason for your extrapolation?

Do people in your field agree that this relationship is right for this chemical (or whatever)?

Who in the population does it apply to? What's the extent of the risk? Can you say what it means to individuals?

Is the risk a definite number or rate, or is there a range of possibilities, depending on your assumptions or differing interpretations of your data?

Is the risk cited for current exposure levels, or for some projected future levels? Is the risk based on the amount of contaminated food that an average person eats, or on the large amounts that only some people eat? Are there individual sensitivities?

Are there alternatives to this chemical (or other agent), and what do we know about their risks?

Animal studies – Have animal studies been done on this chemical? Were they long-term studies (such as two-year or longer bioassays for cancer) or short-term (six months or so). Short-term studies yield quick results, but are not as good as long-term studies.

Were studies conducted for mutagenicity and reproductive effects as well as for cancer? How many species were tested? Usually it's mice and rats.

What was the method of exposure? Inhalation? Feeding? Skin exposure (dermal)? Something in our food supply might best be tested by a feeding study; a workplace exposure, by skin exposure. (For more on animal studies, see "Animals as Stand-Ins for Us" in Chapter 6.)

A fit with other findings? – What do other experts think? Are there other studies or conclusions that bear out what you say? Can you cite specific ones that I can look up?

Special statistical situations

Some other things to keep in mind as you ask questions:

Scaling up – Inappropriate scaling can produce two common errors that are made by both journalists and analysts:

- You see 2 or 3 or 20 cases of a disease and assume that the results apply to a larger population. This is the *individualistic fallacy*. Your sample must be large enough, and representative enough, before you may reliably and validly extrapolate.
- You study 10 cities along the Ohio River and find a relationship between water quality and reported bladder cancer. You assume that there is probably a cause-and-effect relationship. And you assume that the same is probably true anyplace with the same water quality, and that individuals or groups of individuals in other cities with similar water quality must be victims of the same problem. You may be engaging in the *ecological fallacy*. If you studied 100 towns with the same kind of water, or did a careful comparison of bladder cancer patients with comparable controls, you might find that something entirely different caused the cancers.

Another way of counting – One more term that you may encounter in some types of studies: *nonparametric methods*. These are methods of examining data that do not rely on a numerical distribution. As a result, they don't allow a few very large or very small or very wild numbers to run away with the analysis. *Example*: Using just plus or minus signs rather than specific counts for reactions to a substance or a medical treatment. You count up and compare the number of pluses and minuses. Or you might group your counts by rank from least to greatest.

These methods can sometimes be valuable – when used with care. Ask the researcher why this approach was used; look for a reasoned answer.

Notes

1. In this chapter, we drew substantially on the presentations, and often the words, of Dr. Michael Greenberg at Rutgers University and Dr. Peter Montague at Princeton University at science writers' symposiums. Cass Peterson of the *Washington Post* and others added their inputs. Some of their comments also were helpful for the next chapter.

2. Peter Montague checklist, quoted in Cohn, *Reporting on Risk*, p. 38, as well as from the science writers' symposiums.
3. http://web.mit.edu/jsterman/www/Skeptic%27s_Guide.html
4. This edition of *News & Numbers* was going to press as the nuclear plant failures at the Fukushima Daiichi plant in Japan were unfolding; hence they are not accounted for in this section.
5. Barbara S. Hulka, "When Is the Evidence for 'No Association' Sufficient?" (editorial), *Journal of the American Medical Association* 252, no. 1 (July 6, 1984): 811–12.
6. Kenneth Rothman, Boston University, quoted in Gina Kolata, "Cell Phone Studies See No Link to Brain Cancer," *New York Times*, December 20, 2000. Other information is from this and other news reports.
7. "How Lobbyists Play the Numbers Game," *Newsweek*, February 12, 1990.
8. Baruch Fischhoff, "Reporting on Environmental and Health Risks," in *NewsBackgrounder*, Foundation for American Communications.
9. Dorothy Nelkin, background paper in *Science in the Streets: Report of the Twentieth Century Fund Task Force on the Communication of Scientific Risk* (New York: Priority Press, 1984).
10. Gary D. Friedman, personal communication.

10

Writing About Risks

You can drown in the middle of a lake with an average *depth of four feet.*

Author unknown

People love to read about the risks that they worry about.

They worry about their risk of catching the latest disease going around – or a sinister one that might come.

They cringe as they watch risk-loving kids whiz down the street on new-fangled skateboards, and would relish reading about how this fad is affecting emergency room business. Then with awe, they marvel at the risks faced by our astronauts each time the shuttle flies.

They fret about possible risks from a strange smell in the air, or a worrisome taste in the water, or the puzzling radon gas that invades some homes. And they hope to learn more.

They grimace about the unknowns in assessing the risks from terrorism. And after Katrina, they know that they should worry more about other awesome risks of nature.

Numbers help us evaluate and write about the innumerable risks that make news. That's why AIDS and other ills, medication side effects, environmental concerns, and other risks have been discussed throughout this book. This new chapter ties together, and adds much to, these important discussions – with tips from top reporters and others. Some of the tips

News & Numbers: A Writer's Guide to Statistics, Third Edition. Victor Cohn and Lewis Cope with Deborah Cohn Runkle.
© 2012 Victor Cohn and Lewis Cope. Published 2012 by Blackwell Publishing Ltd.

apply more to one type of risk than another, but most have broad applications. And some also may help in writing about subjects beyond risks.[1]

Reader-Friendly Writing

Six basics:

1. **Personalize the risk numbers.** *Example*: If a state's homicide rate is "8.0 per 100,000 per year," you can say "one person in every 12,500 will be a homicide victim this year, if current rates continue."
2. **Put a human feel on the risks when you can.** Jim Detjen, who was a top reporter for the *Philadelphia Inquirer*, says: "Write about things in a way your readers can relate to. Don't just say so many parts per million of sulfur dioxide are going into the air; explain how those levels can trigger asthmatic attacks among the sick and elderly."[2]
3. **Put a human face on the risk when appropriate.** Many stories can be enhanced by interviewing people who already have become ill or injured, or who are at high risk for that happening. Detjen again, speaking about environmental victims but with advice that applies to others as well: "You don't need to sensationalize. An accurate picture is often alarming enough."
4. **Add a real-people touch – with added insights.** Sometimes the people "who really know what's going on" aren't the conventional experts, Detjen says. On pollution, you may be able to add to your story by talking with fishermen, seamen, foresters, or airline pilots. For an article on road rage or other traffic risks, we suggest that you talk to cab drivers or commercial truck drivers, who see it all every day and night.
5. **Make comparisons, but with care** – *Examples*: How does the risk from the disease that you're writing about compare with some other, well-known illness? For example, how does the risk of a worrisome flu "pandemic" – such as H1N1 – compare to the risks from the usual seasonal flu? How does some serious occupational risk compare with the chances of dying in a traffic accident? How does any risk compare to something else that people can easily relate to?

    But caution: Someone can make almost any risk seem small by comparing it to cigarette smoking, which has been linked to about 400,000 deaths a year in the United States.

Or you may be told, "It's *so safe* that you are at greater risk of being struck by lightning." Well, lightning strikes aren't that uncommon. And this reminds us how increased exposure can increase some risks: A diehard golfer who plays in a thundershower may discover that the lightning risk isn't as small as he might have wished.

6. **Help people when you can.** *A few of many possible examples:* When writing about the lung cancer risk from high levels of invisible radon gas that invades some homes, you can tell people how pipes, fans, and other methods can be used to make their homes safer from this naturally occurring, radioactive gas. For an article about the risk of various illnesses or injuries, you can provide key prevention or risk-reduction tips.

For many stories, you can offer your readers or viewers a web site or other source for more information. But make sure that the information is worth passing on – which, in the case of a web site, includes trying it out first.

Helpful Numbers

Needed numbers too often are missing in articles about risks. Here are four basics, with a few of many possible examples:

1. **Put a number on a risk** whenever possible. Don't just say the risk is small or great. Will 1 out of every 10 patients who take a particular prescription pill have a specific side effect? Or 1-in-100, or 1-in-100,000 risk, or what?
2. **Keep time in mind.** The average driver faces a 1-in-1,000 risk of having a specific type of accident, safety-researchers tell us in a news release. But is that the odds *per year*? Or over the *5 years studied*? Or the chances of it happening over a *lifetime* of driving?
3. **Use a denominator** when it helps define a risk.

   Fifty students in a school are struck by a viral illness. How many students go to that school?

   One hundred people develop a life-threatening side effect after taking a new drug. How many people took the drug? In some cases: How many of these people meet the medical criteria that put them at greatest risk? For example, one widely used drug on the market increased the risk of heart attacks, but close study showed that the risk was greatest for patients with preexisting heart conditions.

4. **Prefer ranges** over worst-case figures. "As many as ..." leads are too common – such as "As many as a jillion could be killed." There may be a good enough reason to use such leads in some cases, but high–low ranges tell more. And surely, don't make the reader wait until the 22nd paragraph for the low number.

Risk-rating numbers

Relative risk and absolute risk are two calculations used to rate risks. They are quite different – yet both are quite important.

Relative risk compares two different groups of people, such as smokers and nonsmokers.

Another example: People exposed to a particular chemical in the workplace are five times more likely to develop a particular lung problem *compared with people who are not exposed*, a study concludes. The relative risk is 5.

Absolute risk tells you what to expect over a given time period. It can tell you, for example, the "number of cases *per 10,000 population per year*," or variations on numbers like that.

Take the workplace example cited above: An absolute risk calculation shows that you can expect "35 additional cases of this lung problem ailment per 10,000 workers per year." In all, 20,000 people work with this problem-causing chemical at various plants across the country. So about 70 workers will be affected over the next 12 months – or until effective protective steps can be taken.

An important principle: In total lives affected, a small increased risk for a common illness can be more important than a large increased risk for a rare illness.

Example: A *relative risk* calculation shows that a new prescription pill triples the risk of a person developing a particular kidney problem. But an *absolute risk* calculation shows that this kidney problem is so rare in the first place that tripling the risk will cause only two additional cases per 10,000 pill-users per year.[3]

Relative risk is often easiest for people to relate to. And it makes some possible risks show up like a sore thumb (or if the numbers aren't that clear, like a sore little finger). But absolute risks can show the actual health or other impact. When offered one, you may want to ask for the other as well.

Small numbers – A relative risk of 1.5 can be expressed as a 50 percent increase in risk. *But caution:* A small relative risk number may or may not signal a problem, given the limited reliability of observation, chance, and other possible variables. A relative risk of less than 2.0 is a signal for a reporter to ask more questions for assurance that the risk is real, some experts suggest. (See Chapter 7, "Putting Numbers on Risks.")

Of course, there also can be uncertainty when any calculations must be based on limited or questionable data. See the item on uncertainty in the checklist later in this chapter.

The Human Equations

Let math expert Douglas Hofstadter stir your thinking:

> Can you imagine how we would react if someone said … "Hey, everybody! I've come up with a really nifty invention. Unfortunately it has a minor defect. Every [18 years or so], it will wipe out about as many Americans as the population of San Francisco!" That's what automobile accidents do.[4]

But who wants to go back to the horse and buggy? The convenience of cars outweighs their risk, virtually all Americans would agree.

To write well about risks, we need to understand how our readers think about risks. Some common risk perceptions make good sense – but, frankly, others don't. So to expand on the brief discussion in the last chapter, let's look at seven things that push people's worry buttons:[5]

1. **People typically worry most about the risks that are imposed on them,** rather than those that they take voluntarily. They worry about an industrial plant's smokestack emissions as they speed down the highway with their seat belts unbuckled. They worry about overhead power lines as they start a day of downhill skiing or bungee-jumping. This is understandable – up to a point. Nobody likes to be put in danger, and life should allow for some risky pleasures.

   But the biggest risks that people face tend to be *self-imposed* ones: Smoking, overeating, drug abuse, and drunk driving. So Pogo was right when he said "we have met the enemy and he is us," veteran science writer Cristine Russell points out in *A Field Guide for Science Writers*.[6]

2. **There's the related I'm-in-control factor.** After a big airliner crash, some people may decide to drive to their next vacation – even though experts tell us it's safer to fly than drive.

Of course, you can lower your risk when you drive by slowing down. But many people don't.

3. **People tend to worry more about man-made risks** than natural ones – which is one more reason that they worry a lot about environmental threats. The good news: It's often easier to reduce the human-generated risks. The concern: We need to be prepared not only for hurricanes, as Katrina taught the nation, but for other weather worries such as tornadoes, flooding, and blizzards.

4. **People worry more when risks are new and the uncertainty is high.** Remember the anxiety in the early days of AIDS? *Today:* When will terrorists strike next? What's the chance of another anthrax attack? Another bomb placed in a parked car?

5. **Some risks are mysteriously threatening,** which heightens concern. Strange smells in the air can be alarming – at least until explained. And any cancer is alarming to some people, while clusters of cancer cases are alarming to many. But cancer clusters may be due to chance alone. (See Chapter 7, "Confusing Clusters.")

6. **The surprise factor can shock us.** People accept that prescription drugs carry risks. But many people may feel blindsided by cases such as the arthritis drug Vioxx, where a big heart risk was disclosed only after years of widespread use.

   To avoid surprise, industrial firms can be upfront in dealing with people's concerns about what they're doing and planning to do. Some companies don't think this way. But as journalists, we can.

7. **Personal fears can add to worries.** Even beyond the obvious difference between a skin rash and death, people worry more about some health consequences than about others. For example, some people fear severe, permanent brain damage as much as death itself. And the risks of fates like shark attacks can be so chilling that we shiver even thinking about them.

Knowledge of these seven risk-perception principles can help us as journalists in three ways: We can better spot *what* is likely to be most newsworthy to the public. We can write better stories by knowing *when* and *how* we need to stir people's thinking and calm some fears. And we can add depth to some of our writings by explaining *why* people think about specific risks as they do.

Here's a risk story that may leave you scratching your head:

More and more bicycle riders – adults and children alike – began wearing helmets for safety's sake. But then bike-riding head injuries *rose* by about

50 percent. An insightful *New York Times* article looked at several possibilities, such as whether there are enough safe places for biking. But risk experts quoted by the *Times* suggested a more intriguing explanation: Too many riders felt too safe wearing the helmets – and then took too many risks. Bike-safety experts now know how to target their prevention messages.[7]

A Risk-Writer's Checklist

Three basics to consider as you write:

- **Averages** – It's not the average amount of a toxic chemical in the air that's most important. It's the amount downwind – where people are breathing it. *Also*: Different workers at a company may be exposed to different amounts of a suspect chemical; *the* average overall risk isn't *an* average for each individual worker. (See Chapter 9, "Let the Questions Fly.")
- **Individual vulnerability** – Children, asthmatics, or people in other groups may be most affected by particular chemicals, illnesses, or other threats.
- **Prevention** – Stay alert to the possibilities of risk reduction.

Watch your language:

- **Uncertainties.** If risk studies are based on only limited data, or have other weaknesses, say so. If no one knows the answer to a key question, say so. When appropriate, don't hesitate to say "might," or use other qualifiers such as "some experts believe."
- **Relative safety.** We hear of safe drugs, safe cars, environmental safety, safety caps. Then comes a manufacturer's recall of cars, for safety's sake. Or some medication side effect warning. Or some other alert or recall. Things are seldom completely safe. Often we should say, "This means relatively safe." And then we should try to indicate the degree of safety or risk.

Consider for your writings, as applicable:

- **Risks versus benefits** – Who bears the risks? Who gets the benefits? *And a related cost–benefit question*: Who pays for what? (See Chapter 9, "Let the Questions Fly" and "Risk–Benefit Assessments.")
- **The need for other numbers** – To make a problem sound smaller or larger, you may be offered an annual death toll or a lifetime toll.

130

Other figures also can confuse an issue. Ask for all the numbers that you need. (See Chapter 9, "Testing the Evidence.")

- **The risk of over-reacting** – *Example*: When risks of side effects from some prescription drug are in the news, doctors sometimes caution patients *not* to stop taking it – at least until they can be put on a substitute medicine. So when appropriate: Ask experts not only what people should do – but what they shouldn't do.

To avoid jumping to wrong conclusions, remember:

- **Association alone doesn't prove causation** – *One of many possible examples*: The chemical in a workplace may or may not be the cause of illnesses there. More study is needed. (See Chapter 3, "Cause–Effect.")
- **The healthy-worker effect** – Workers in general tend to be in better health than the overall population. So just because a group of workers is in "above-average health" doesn't prove that there is no health risk lurking in their midst. More study is needed. (See Chapter 3, "Workers, Placebos, and Surveys.")
- **Cluster confusion** – As mentioned above, relatively large numbers of cancer cases in a town or neighborhood may be due to chance alone. The same can happen with birth defects. More study is needed. (See Chapter 7, "Confusing Clusters.")

Three thoughts about time, for use in your stories as helpful or needed:

- **Long latency period** (the time-bomb effect). Some types of cancer and certain other ills don't develop for many years after exposure starts. This can lull people into a false sense of security. *Examples*: Smoking and lung cancer, and risks from workplace exposure to asbestos.
- **Length-of-threat time.** *One of many possible examples*: Experts estimate that it will take three years to clean up a contaminated worksite.
- **Exposure time.** *One example of many possible*: A serious side effect is found for a drug, but only in patients who have taken it for at least 12 months.

And Looking Ahead

- **What now?** *In typical cases*: Who's planning to do what? When? What more might be done? *Sometimes*: What might be the risk of delay, or inaction? *Always consider*: What else should the public know?

131

Tips that Reach Well Beyond Risks

Three tips from risk-writing experts that apply to all areas of reporting:

1. **Read. Learn. Cultivate long-term sources.** These people will be far easier to tap, and far more forthcoming, once they know you've done some homework.
2. **Don't be afraid to challenge an expert.** Dr. Dorothy Nelkin at Cornell University says, "The most serious problem" in reporting on risk may be the reluctance of some journalists to challenge their sources and "those who use the authority of science to shape the public view." Maintain "the spirit of independent, critical inquiry that has guided good investigation in other areas."[8]
3. **"Follow up, follow up, follow up,"** says Detjen. In writing about various problems, report what, if anything, gets done. And for research, follow up to see if early leads – and hopes or fears – are confirmed.

Notes

1. We again extend appreciation to the experts who helped with the previous chapter. Their comments provided risk information that was helpful for this chapter, too. Also, this chapter's checklist section has brief summaries of points covered elsewhere in this book, with references to those earlier pages. Source notes are with the reports in earlier chapters.
2. Tips from Jim Detjen, here and elsewhere in this chapter, are from a talk at CASW seminars "Public Health and the Environment," and from his comments in Cohn, *Reporting on Risk*.
3. Adapted from another example in *A Field Guide for Science Writers*, 2nd edn., eds. Deborah Blum, Mary Knudson, and Robin Marantaz Henig (New York: Oxford University Press, 2006), p. 253. This is the official guidebook of the National Association of Science Writers, written by a large cast of science writers. Cristine Russell wrote the risk chapter.
4. Douglas R. Hofstadter, *Mathematical Themas* (New York: Basic Books, 1985).
5. In part, from David Ropeik, "Journalists Can Be Seduced by Aspects of Risks," Nieman Reports, Winter 2002, and Don Colburn, Newhouse News Service, article on risk perceptions, December 2001.
6. Russell, *A Field Guide for Science Writers*, 254.
7. Julian E. Barnes, "A Bicycling Mystery: Head Injuries Pilling Up," *New York Times*, July 29, 2001.
8. Dorothy Nelkin, background paper in *Science in the Streets: Report of the Twentieth Century Fund Task Force on the Communication of Scientific Risk* (New York: Priority Press, 1984).

11

Polls

A president cannot always be popular.

Harry Truman

People eagerly await, and may be influenced by, the polls that probe hot-button issues and hard-fought election races.

Then different polls come up with widely different views of the public's opinions on some topics, such as electronic eavesdropping and stem cell research.

And remember how the exit polls on Election Day 2004 told us that John Kerry was whipping George Bush in key states?

We'll get back to those problems as we move through this chapter. But let's start with a classic case example that reminds us of two prime no-no's of science-based polling:

Political gadfly Ross Perot, founder of the Reform Party, asked in a mail-in poll: "Should laws be passed to eliminate all possibilities of special interests giving huge sums of money to candidates?" Ninety-nine percent of the people who responded said *yes*.

Then the prestigious polling firm Yankelovich and Partners asked the very same question to a scientifically based, national sampling of Americans. Now 80 percent said *yes*.

News & Numbers: A Writer's Guide to Statistics, Third Edition. Victor Cohn and Lewis Cope with Deborah Cohn Runkle.
© 2012 Victor Cohn and Lewis Cope. Published 2012 by Blackwell Publishing Ltd.

Finally the polling firm asked a more neutral version of the question to another scientifically based sampling of people across the nation: "Should laws be passed to prohibit interest groups from contributing to campaigns, or do groups have a right to contribute to the candidate they support?" Those in favor of prohibiting contributions dropped to 40 percent.[1]

Perot's poll had two big problems: First, his poll was published in a magazine and was dependent on who read the magazine and then which readers chose to mail in their answers. Thus the people polled were self-selected – and not a required random sampling of voters. Second, Perot's question was biased – or, if you prefer a nonscientific term, *loaded*.

Although this chapter focuses on the political and opinion polls that regularly make headlines, other uses of polling provide estimates of national unemployment, car seat-belt use, immunization rates, and many other things. These studies are often called "surveys" rather than polls. But good polling techniques are needed in these endeavors, too. So let's walk through …

The Principles of Polling

The four basics:

1. **Random sampling can make 1 = 200,000.** In a typical national poll, about 1,000 people may be interviewed to get results showing what 200 million American adults think about political candidates or issues. That means that the poll is using the response of each person interviewed to represent what approximately 200,000 people think. The principle is the same for a state or regional poll, although the numbers will vary.

   You can't just interview the first 1,000 people who pass you on the street. They aren't representative of a larger population, but rather represent the people who live or work or shop in that neighborhood. To make a poll work, the selection of people polled must be a random sampling that can represent the characteristics of all Americans, or some other population group. For example, if you wanted to know what Hispanics think about a law passed in Arizona, you'd want a random sample of Hispanics.

   Here's how the highly respected Minnesota Poll in the Minneapolis–St. Paul *StarTribune* explained this part of its polling technique to its readers: "A random-digit-dial telephone sample of 1,001 adult

Minnesotans" was used. "Results for the poll were weighted for age, gender and education to make sure that the sample reflected ... census estimates for Minnesota's adult population."[2]

Pollsters point to a random-sampling problem in the Bush–Kerry exit polling, as we'll see in the case histories section.

TV-watching alert: When a TV show asks viewers to phone in their responses to an "instant poll," they'll often say "this isn't a scientific poll." That's sure true. The people watching the show are a self-selected group – who probably favor the political bent of the TV show. And those who care most about the issue are the ones most likely to pick up the phone to "vote." That's not random sampling. So you can't count on these findings, any more than those of a magazine's mail-in poll.

2. **The size of a poll determines its margin of sampling error.** The more people who are polled, the smaller the margin of sampling error. A *New York Times* poll used admirable candor to tell readers about a poll that interviewed 900 adults:

In theory, in 19 cases out of 20, the results based on such samples will differ by no more than 3 percentage points in either direction from that which would have been obtained by interviewing all adult New Yorkers. For smaller groups, the potential error is greater. For all whites, plus or minus 4 percentage points. For all blacks, it is plus or minus 7 points. In addition to sampling error, the practical difficulties of conducting any survey of public opinion may introduce other sources of error into the poll.[3]

This is about the best explanation of the uncertainties of polling that we've seen.

When it's too close to call, a poll should admit it. If candidate A is leading candidate B, but the poll's results are still within its margin of sampling error, the news report should clearly say so and should caution against concluding that one candidate leads another. The same applies to polls that probe issues or attitudes.

Think of it this way: If you have a thermometer that can't detect temperature differences as small as .1 degree, you would be wrong to say that 82.1 degrees is hotter than 82.0 degrees. Your measuring instrument just isn't that good. Same with polls.

3. **Fair questions are vital.**

Poll questions shouldn't unfairly tilt toward a particular answer – much less lean as far as Perot's question did.

But sometimes even fair-minded wording choices can affect polls' responses. *The stem cell and eavesdropping polls are good examples, as we'll see in the case histories section.*

Also, all poll questions should be clear enough to avoid confusing answers.

Advocacy alert: Extra vigilance is needed for polls commissioned by an advocacy or political organization, or other special interest group. *That also was a factor in some of the stem cell polling.* And it was true in evaluating and reporting on scientific studies (See Chapter 3).

4. **A poll is only a snapshot, taken at one point in time.** At best, polls can only tell what people are thinking at the time they're polled. People's views often change over time. Candidates often roam up and down in public favor over time. For this reason, tracking polls are often conducted, which follow the same people over a period of time to detect trends in voting decisions.

   Intervening-events alert: If a poll is taken before a candidate made a serious gaffe, but the poll is not published until afterward, that should be clearly noted. Ditto for all similar intervening events.

   Voter turnout decides some elections. So pollsters ask questions designed to weed out participants who are unlikely to vote on election day. *Examples*: Did you vote in the last election? How interested are you in this election?[4]

Nevertheless, nothing can guarantee that any specific poll will be on target. Pollster Burns W. Roper was once asked the same question that his firm had asked in a poll: How do you assess the accuracy of polls? His response: "Usually accurate."[5]

Case Histories

Bush–Kerry exit polling: random failure

Exit-polling guidelines deal with how interviewers can get a random sampling of voters, such as by interviewing every fifth or sixth voter who walks out of a polling place on Election Day.

But many of the people recruited to do the Bush–Kerry exit polling were relatively young, and this made them more successful in getting Kerry voters to stop for interviews, the chief pollsters for that project now say. This explains why exit polls in some key states overstated voters' support for Kerry, who obviously didn't get the real votes that counted.

For the next election, the pollsters planned to select interviewers from across all age groups – and provide better training.[6]

Eavesdropping and stem cells: the questions

The wiretaps-terrorism issue – News reports in early 2006 disclosed that the federal National Security Agency was conducting warrantless wiretaps of some international communications. Different pollsters came up with quite different conclusions about whether Americans favored or were against what was going on.

"A key distinction appears to be the way pollsters identify the people who might have their email and phone calls monitored as part of an effort to fight terrorism," noted Carl Bialik in his Numbers Guy column for the *Wall Street Journal Online* (wsj.com).

One poll asked if the government should be allowed to intercept calls between "terrorism suspects" overseas and "people living in the United States." Almost two-thirds said *yes*, Bialik noted. But in another poll, a slight majority *opposed* the wiretaps when the question included words like "U.S. citizens living in the United States," and emphasized the lack of a court order.[7]

The stem cell controversy – Medical researchers hope that stem cells from human embryos can be used to treat many different illnesses. But the embryos are destroyed in the process, so some people oppose this on moral grounds.

Although most polls by the news media and other independent organizations have found that a majority of Americans support this type of research, some polls haven't. And the amount of support has varied greatly – from about 45 percent up to about 75 percent.

Again, the wording of the question in the poll can affect whether the result is at the top or bottom of that range. When Alzheimer's, cancer, and other medical problems that might be helped by stem cell therapy are specifically mentioned in the questioning, results tend to be at the top of the range.

In addition to these polls, opponents and proponents of embryonic stem cell therapy have commissioned their own polls. One question in a poll for opponents referred only to "experiments" with "live" embryos. That dropped public support to 24 percent.[8]

Our comments: Both the wiretap-terrorism and the stem cell issues are unusually complex, increasing the chances that different pollsters will ask questions that differ enough to get different results. And that becomes part of the story.

More questions about questions

The Pew Research Center for the People and the Press came up with an innovative test that proves the strong powers of poll-question wording. In a special poll, the center first noted that President Clinton had proposed setting aside about two-thirds of an expected budget surplus to fix the Social Security system. The Pew center poll then …

Asked some people: Should the rest of the budget surplus be used for a tax cut, or should this money "be used to fund new government programs." The results: 60 percent said cut taxes, and only 25 percent said fund new programs. Eleven percent said the money should be used for other purposes.

Asked of another group of people: Should the rest of the surplus be used for a tax cut, or should it be spent "on programs for education, the environment, health care, crime-fighting and military defense." Now only 22 percent said cut taxes, and 69 percent said spend it on the listed programs. Six percent said use the money for other purposes.

(The figures don't add up to 100 percent because some people polled said they didn't know, or didn't want to answer.[9])

Comments: We note, with admiration, that some polls have turned situations like this into even better polls. They use a "double-barreled" questioning approach. For example, they first ask: "What do you think in general …" about government spending (or whatever). Then they ask a second question, "What do you think about …" a specific spending idea (or whatever). And then the poll story can track the intricacies of public thinking about a complex issue – and where people really want their politicians to go.

What's asked first – The order in which questions are asked also may affect the results. If you first ask pointed questions about problems that one candidate is having, you may skew the results of a following how-will-you-vote question.

In a poll at the height of the Cold War in the 1950s, Americans were asked if they thought that the United States should allow "Communist reporters from other countries [to] come in here and send back to their papers the news as they see it." Only 36 percent said *yes*. But the *yes* answers increased to 73 percent when the very same question was preceded by one asking if Russia should admit American reporters.[10]

Ventura and Reagan: explaining the uncertainty

Ventura's body slam – A poll can be right even when it doesn't call the winner.

When ex-pro-wrestler Jesse ("the Body") Ventura was elected Minnesota governor in 1998, readers of the Minneapolis–St. Paul *StarTribune* clearly weren't as surprised as most Americans. Two days earlier, the newspaper's Minnesota Poll was able to tell its readers that although Ventura was still running number three in the three-man race, each contender "has a real chance of claiming the governor's office on election day."

Eight percentage points divided the three candidates, which was more than the margin of sampling error. But the newspaper cited the poll's trend data to show how Ventura was gaining ground in an unusually volatile race. The poll data also showed that many Minnesotans felt Ventura was in tune with them on key issues, indicating that he might get some late-minute converts.

And the poll article said the winner could be determined by which candidate could do the best job of getting his voters to the polls. That's just what Ventura did to win.[11]

Reagan and the ABCs of polling – Within a few weeks in July 1984, five major polls gave President Reagan a lead varying from 1 to 26 points over Walter Mondale. Then in their final, most careful predictions on election eve, seven polls gave the president leads that varied from 10 to 25 points. He won by 18 points. At best, says pollster Richard Wirthlin, polling is an "ABC science, **A**lmost **B**eing **C**ertain," because "we are not dealing with reality directly, but through a mirror darkly clouded."[12]

Polls beyond politics: speed and smoke

The value of polls goes beyond political races and hot-button issues. One of the authors of this book (Cope) used polling as a major part of a five-part series on preventive health care in the *StarTribune* of Minneapolis–St. Paul.

He was able to start one article in the series, "Most Minnesotans buckle up for safety – then speed."

And another article: "Minnesotans are smoking less, but being bothered by other people's smoke more."[13]

Writing and Other Tips

Know when to write "percentage points" rather than "percent."
Rob Daves, former director of the Minnesota Poll at the *StarTribune*, offers these guidelines to make things clear, correct, and consistent:

- Use "percentage points" when you are talking about the differences between percents. For example, if 60 percent of the poll's participants favor candidate A and 40 percent favor candidate B, write it, "Candidate A has a 20 *percentage point* lead over B in the poll." Candidate A *does not* have a 20 percent lead over B.
- Use "percentage points" when you are expressing a margin of sampling error. *Example*: "The poll's margin of sampling error is plus or minus 3 *percentage points*."[14]

Percentage points **and** *percent* **do not mean the same thing.**

Don't magnify a small change from one poll to the next. If the president's approval rating goes from 59 to 58 percent, or one candidate's standing edges up 2 points, it may be worth mentioning. But only if the trend continues is it important.

Put extra confidence in findings when more than one poll – asking approximately the same questions – agrees.

Watch out for picky pointing to selective polls. To quote Robert Samuelson, *Newsweek* economics columnist: "To prove the popularity of [an administration's] tax plan, you cite surveys showing that roughly half of the public favor it, with about a third against. To demonstrate opposition, you cite polls indicating large majorities against specific proposals, such as the elimination of the deduction for local taxes."[15]

Watch out for the "whys" in special-interest polling. This includes polls conducted for companies as well as for advocacy groups and politicians. Even when the questions and the polling methods appear valid, consider (and comment on as necessary): Why was this poll taken? And why at this time?

Watch out for political "push polling." Here's how this pseudo-polling, political telemarketing technique is done:

The telephone caller uses the pretext that he's conducting a poll, but the real purpose is to "sell" – or push – a particular political candidate. The caller does this by presenting false or misleading information about the candidate's opponent or by asking what lawyers call "leading questions," then asking how this will affect voter preference.

The American Association for Public Opinion Research warns that push polling "can easily be confused with real polls," which in turn can "damage the reputation of legitimate polling" and discourage people from participating in proper polls.

For more information

The Minnesota Poll's Daves recommends two Internet sites:

- The web site of the National Council on Public Polls is www.ncpp. org. You can read "20 questions a journalist should ask about poll results" and get other information as well.
- The web site for the American Association for Public Opinion Research, with information about "push polling" and other topics, is www.aapor.org.

Challenges in polls dealing with sex

In 1987, author and social investigator Shere Hite published her third book on men and women in bed and out. Hite's findings – on women's attitudes about men, sex, and personal and marital relationships – launched a flood of news stories and TV talk.

Hite had distributed 100,000 lengthy questionnaires to women in groups of many kinds all over the country. On the basis of 4,500 replies, she reported that 84 percent of the women in her study were dissatisfied with their marital or other intimate relationships. She reported that 78 percent said that they were generally not treated as equals by men and that 70 percent of those married more than five years had had affairs. What followed was more answers of this type, leading to Hite's conclusion that women in general are mainly unhappy with their relationships.

Women in general? Hite said at one point in her book that "no one can generalize" from her findings. Yet she also claimed that her 4,500 respondents were typical of all American women. Critics said her sample was almost certainly heavily weighted with the unhappiest women, those who took the time to answer the lengthy questionnaire. Testing Hite's findings, a *Washington Post*–ABC News polling team questioned a representative sample – representative by proper polling methods – of 767 women and 738 men across the nation. That poll found that 93 percent of the married and single women said they were satisfied with their relationships, 81 percent said they were treated as equals most of the time, and only 7 percent reported affairs.

That survey, like most surveys, was conducted by phone. Hite said women would not be candid to a telephone caller. Jeff Alderman, ABC polling director, replied, "Over the phone, people will say things to us they wouldn't say to a neighbor. We've never had any indication they lie."

But Richard Morin, *Washington Post* polling director, conceded that these sunny results should be interpreted with some care too, since "telephone surveys like this might be expected to overstate satisfaction with personal relationships, and understate, to a significantly greater degree, the extent of socially unacceptable behavior such as adultery."[16]

Who was closer to the truth? We don't know.

Snowballs and Focus Groups

Snowball samples – Reporters occasionally borrow a page from polling, without claiming to have a scientifically accurate poll. They interview a dozen, maybe many more, supposedly randomly chosen people in a community to get a general feeling of attitudes about an election, about an issue, or about a controversy. An experienced editor offers his concerns about this practice:

They'll make this common mistake: They'll ask somebody – somebody picked at random, perhaps – a question, but then take *that* person's recommendation on the next person to talk to, because the first person has said, "I'll tell you somebody else who knows a lot about that."

At that point they no longer have a random sample. I think the expression for this is a *snowball sample*. What made me aware of it was that a couple of professors did a survey of Vietnamese refugees in this country, asking about their treatment in refugee camps back in Vietnam. The professors interviewed one family, then that family knew another family, and so on. They soon realized they were getting only one story and changed their methodology. It makes you realize how easily you can skew things, even inadvertently.[17]

A statistician adds: True enough and worth guarding against, but snowball sampling can be a good way to collect information about a particular class of persons with the same interests or problems. Just don't confuse them with a representative sample of a broader population.

Focus groups – Political candidates and business firms often use focus groups to gauge public opinion. Typically, a small group of people is brought together for an in-depth interview by a trained moderator. The moderator uses follow-up questions to probe deeper than a poll would allow. And since it's done in person rather than over the phone, the people being interviewed can be shown a company's new product or a planned TV ad.

This approach may uncover a surprise finding that a pollster would not have thought to ask about. A good focus group moderator is much like a good reporter conducting a group interview.

But caution: Focus groups aren't scientific polls. They are too small to serve as a representative sampling of the public. There's no way to know how widespread the group's opinions apply. And when a reporter is told that a political party's or a company's focus group has found something that favors candidate X or company Y, the reporter can't readily tell whether the focus group discussion was tilted in some way.

Notes

1. Daniel Goleman, in-depth report on polling techniques, "Pollsters Enlist Psychologists in Quest for Unbiased Results," *New York Times*, September 7, 1993.
2. "How the Poll Was Conducted," *StarTribune* of Minneapolis–St. Paul, November 28, 1999.
3. "How the Poll Was Conducted," *New York Times*, January 9, 1987.
4. These examples, and some general observations for this chapter, are based on an interview with Rob Daves, director of the Minnesota Poll at the *StarTribune* of Minneapolis–St. Paul.
5. Burns Roper, quoted in "Private Opinions on Public Opinion: Question Is, What Is the Question?," *New York Times*, August 24, 1994.
6. Jacques Steinberg, "Study Cites Human Failings in Election Day Poll System," *New York Times*, January 20, 2005; and Will Lester, Associated Press dispatch on polling, May 14, 2005.
7. Carl Binlik, "Sometimes in Polling, It's All in the Question," in his Numbers Guy column, *Wall Street Journal Online*, February 7, 2006, and other news reports.
8. Adam Clymer, "The Unbearable Lightness of Public Opinion Polls," *New York Times*, July 22, 2001, and other reports.
9. Associated Press report on the Pew Research Center poll, July 22, 1999.
10. Goleman, "Pollsters Enlist Psychologists."
11. Dane Smith, "The Stretch Run: It's Up for Grabs," *StarTribune* of Minneapolis–St. Paul, November 1, 1998.

12. Richard Wirthlin, quoted in "Public Opinion Polls: Are They Science or Art?" *Los Angeles Times – Washington Post* News Service, August 27, 1984.

13. Lewis Cope, "Save Your Life," five-part series in *StarTribune* of Minneapolis–St. Paul; each Thursday, October 8 through November 5, 1992.

14. The Minnesota Poll's Daves offers more detailed information on percentage points, and other help on writing and editing poll articles, in *Contemporary Editing,* by Cecilia Friend, Don Challenger, and Katherine C. McAdams, (Lincolnwood, Ill.: NTC/Contemporary Publishing Company), pp. 354–55.

15. Robert Samuelson, "The Joy of Statistics," *Newsweek,* November 4, 1985.

16. Shere Hite, *Women and Love: A Cultural Revolution in Progress* (New York: Alfred A. Knopf, 1987); Sally Squires, "Modem Couples Say They're Happy Together," *Washington Post,* October 27, 1987; David Streitfeld, "Shere Hite and the Trouble With Numbers," *Washington Post,* November 10, 1987; "Hite Lacks Depth, Says Rival Poll," *New York Daily News,* October 29, 1987; Arlie Russell Hochschild, "Why Can't a Man Be More Like a Woman?" *New York Times Book Review,* November 15, 1987; "Men Aren't Her Only Problem," *Newsweek,* November 23, 1987.

17. Ralph Kinney Bennett, *Reader's Digest,* interview with author.

12

Statistical Savvy
for Many Types of News

Democracy is the worst form of government, except all those other forms that have been tried from time to time.

Sir Winston Churchill

Learn how the Lake Wobegon Effect allows most schools to claim they're "above average."

See why many police departments are "blinding" the lineups they run for eyewitnesses to finger suspects.

Check out the criticism of a study that called for families to eat dinner together to reduce drug abuse.

Consider how a missing number led to misleading information about the costs to taxpayers of three sports stadiums.

But first, let's take a quick glance at the bigger picture:

Government officials and others are continually telling us "we have learned that ..." or "statistics show that ..." or "the computer shows ..." This is followed by words that depend on numbers.

There is every reason to apply some good-sense tests to all such statements by politicians, government officials, economists, salespersons, sports coaches, and others. We must identify the good and thwart any attempts to pull statistics over our eyes. In addition to using various tests discussed throughout this book, we should be alert for some ...

News & Numbers: A Writer's Guide to Statistics, Third Edition. Victor Cohn and Lewis Cope with Deborah Cohn Runkle.
© 2012 Victor Cohn and Lewis Cope. Published 2012 by Blackwell Publishing Ltd.

Statistical Shenanigans

Statistician Nancy Lyon Spruill, writing in the *Washington Post*, warned against what she described as politicians' tricks – although they aren't confined to politicians:[1]

The everything-is-going-up statistic. More people are employed, or more people are getting support payments, or whatever. Correct, because there are more people than ever. A more informative statistic would be the employment or unemployment *rate* or the portion of the population getting welfare payments.

Another example: A Department of Agriculture official once hailed the finding that pork exports had tripled in a two-month period. Further analysis, by others, showed that prior to this report few pork products were being exported. Anytime "you start ... with a small base, the percentage increase is going to be large."[2]

Another example: If the literacy rate in some poor country is only 2 percent, doubling it still means that the country has an abysmally low number of literate citizens.

The best-foot statistic. Selecting whatever number best supports a case, as in choosing between median and mean family income. If the rich get richer and the poor get poorer, the median might stay unchanged. If a few get richer, the mean income will be dragged up, even if incomes for most families remain unchanged. And if a few get much, much richer, the mean income can go up even if there's an increase in poverty.

Another example: Picking the best-sounding year (or years) for comparison. To show an increase in family income, you can compare the prosperous present with a recession year. Things would look different if your comparison year was an average year.

The "gee-whiz" or half-truth statistic. *Example*: Using numbers for only part of the population. If the unemployment rate isn't as high as you'd like it to be, talk about the rate for teenagers or the rate in industrial states, which are generally higher than for the rest of the population.

Another example: To deplore defense spending, tell how increases in defense spending have increased the national debt; don't mention how increases in domestic and entitlement spending have done the same thing.

The coincidence statistic. Whoever is in office is blamed for a recession, though economists can't agree on the cause. Whoever is in office also takes credit for a boom, though.

There's also the meaningless statistic. *Fortune* writer Daniel Seligman, in an article titled, "We're Drowning in Phony Statistics," offered this example:[3] A New York City mayor once said that the "overall cleanliness of the streets has risen to 85 percent," up from 56 percent five years earlier. By what objective criteria? Neither the mayor nor his aides could cite any (although it might have been possible to develop some).

The antidotes for these offenses:

- **Ask for *all* the numbers** that you feel you need.
- **Calculate rates of change** from a sensible base. Then look at changes over a long enough time to feel confident in a trend.
- **Ask often, "How do you know?"**

In Other Types of News

Let's move on to examples of numbers and related statistical concepts that are in the news (with some take-home messages in **boldface**):

Education: The Lake Wobegon Effect[4]

It's a result that any high-school math student would question: Studies show that most school districts across the nation report that their students score above the national average on standardized tests, the *New York Times* reported.

How could so many schools beat the average? Cheating has been reported in a few schools. More often, school officials may switch from one form of test to another to get the good scores they crave, the *New York Times* article said.[5] With the recent emphasis on accountability called for in the No Child Left Behind and other education initiatives, many school districts are reporting progress following a change in tests. Further, national comparisons are difficult because the states don't use the same test.

The results have been nicknamed the Lake Wobegon Effect. The reference is to author Garrison Keillor's fictional Minnesota community, where the women are strong, the men good-looking, and the children are all above average.

And it doesn't end with schools. There are so many health and other statistics that a city, state, company, or advocacy group can find *some* way to show how safe, healthy or just-plain-great it is.

The better something sounds, the deeper you may need to probe.

Police: *"blinding" the lineups*

You know the drill from TV cop shows: The eyewitness to a crime picks the "bad guy" out of a police lineup, which includes the suspect alongside several other people.

The trouble is, DNA testing has revealed that mistaken identity occurs more often than once thought. So how can the police make their lineups more reliable?

Many psychologists and other experts recommend that police adopt "blinding" and other scientific safeguards to reduce the risk of any unintentional bias. A growing number of police departments have adopted this new approach, even though critics maintain that they now have evidence that the old way works best.

Here's what the scientific approach calls for:

- The police officer conducting the lineup should not know which person is the suspect. This "blinding" reduces the risk that the officer will unintentionally steer the eyewitness' choice.
- The eyewitness should view the people in the lineup one at a time, not as a group. This allows the witness to concentrate on whether he or she actually saw the person, not on the one who might look the most like the perpetrator.
- The people in the lineup should share some physical characteristics with the suspect. For example, if the suspect is tall, the others in the lineup shouldn't be short.
- And even before those steps are taken, the officer should caution the witness that the suspect might not be in the lineup. This removes any undue pressure on the witness to make an ID.

The new approach has passed extensive tests in research settings. But in a Chicago real-cases study, police concluded that the old way did better in getting eyewitnesses to identify the criminal suspects rather than innocent people in the lineups. Promoters of the new approach insist that the Chicago study was flawed: The old-way ("unblinded") police officers could have influenced the eyewitnesses' choices. Around and around the controversy goes. Please stay tuned.[6]

Story idea: What do police in your city do? What do defense lawyers say about it?

Family life: who eats at home?

A public service TV ad featuring former First Lady Barbara Bush urged families to eat dinner together as a way to help keep youngsters drug-free. The dining advice was based on an anti-drug organization's telephone survey of teenagers. It "found" that the more often youngsters ate dinner with their families, the less was their risk for abusing drugs.

Carl Bialik, who writes the Numbers Guy column for the *Wall Street Journal Online* (wsj.com), cautioned that "before the government takes its war on drugs to the family kitchen, a close look at the study is warranted."

Bialik said the study didn't "account for age – a key failing. You might be unsurprised to learn that 17-year-olds are more likely to use drugs than 12-year-olds. Older teens are also the ones most likely to eat dinner away from their families."[7] In other words, both eating away from one's family and taking drugs may be correlated with the factor of age. Further, when kids are on drugs, they may be less likely to eat with their families because of other anti-social behavior. In other words, the authors of the study may have wrongly assumed what came first.

Be skeptical of simple solutions for big problems and be skeptical of ...

Religion: faith and health

Various studies have found evidence that people who are religiously devout tend to be healthier than average. Don't jump to any conclusion.

"The reason remains far from clear," writes the *Washington Post*'s Rob Stein. But he offered a spectrum of *possibilities* to consider:

"Healthy people may be more likely to join churches. The pious may lead more wholesome lifestyles. Churches, synagogues and mosques may help people take better care of themselves. The quiet meditation and incantations of praying, or the comfort of being prayed for, appears to lower blood pressure, reduce stress hormones, slow the heart rate and have other potentially beneficial effects."[8]

Additionally, the frequent social contact that accompanies attendance at a church, synagogue, or mosque may at least partially account for the good health enjoyed by religious people.

Faithfully consider all possible explanations.

9/11 and Katrina: the changing tolls

After the two airliners with terrorists at the controls crashed into New York City's World Trade Center in 2001, officials first estimated that about 6,300 people had died. Over time, the tragedy's death toll was reduced to about 4,500, then to 2,801, and finally to about 2,750.[9]

While the 9/11 toll is still horrific, it's a reminder that it's not unusual for death tolls to fall in various disasters.

Some worst-case estimates of deaths in Hurricane Katrina, which struck New Orleans and the Gulf Coast, came down – although some washed-away bodies may never be found. Early death "counts" in train accidents and other tragedies often have to be lowered.

Some missing people simply turn up. Two similar names on a fatality list may turn out to be the same person. And dismemberment of some bodies confuses counting. So ask the officials doing the counting:

How sure are you? How did you reach your count?

Sports: slumps and dunks

"The species *homo sapiens* has a powerful propensity to believe that one can find a pattern even when there is no pattern to be found," when random variability or chance produces what only seems to be a pattern. So writes Dr. Julian L. Simon, an economist at the University of Maryland.[10]

Take baseball, he says. A generally good hitter strikes out three or four consecutive times at bat. The coach then declares a "slump" and pulls him out of the lineup. But studies show that short-term performance in most sports varies in the same way that a run of random numbers of coin flips varies. Similarly, it's been shown that a basketball player's chance of making a basket on each try is unaffected by whether he made or missed the previous shot.

There are indeed long-term trends in sports. A good player can become a poor or aging one. But beware of short-term predictions – in sports, economics, and other fields. As one statistician put it, "Even though there may be real trends in a system, many systems inherently have a very large random component which over short terms may obscure the long-term trends."[11]

Reporters love to make predictions. Sometimes too much.

Your pocketbook: ads and stocks

Robert Hooke, the statistician and author, warns us about ads that say: "Independent laboratory tests show that no other leading product is more effective than ours." His translation: "A [purposely] small test was run among the leading products, and no significant difference was observed among the products tested ... There are people around who can make good news for themselves out of anything."[12]

Darrell Huff, author of the small 1954 book *How to Lie with Statistics*, adds this advertising shenanigan:[13]

"If you can't prove what you want to prove, demonstrate something else and pretend that they are the same thing ... You can't prove that your nostrum cures colds, but you can publish a sworn laboratory report that half an ounce of the stuff killed 31,108 germs in a test tube ... It is not up to you ... to point out that an antiseptic that works well in a test tube may not perform in the human throat ... [And] don't confuse the issue by telling what kind of germ you killed."

Huff also tells of a juice extractor that was widely advertised as one that "extracts 26 percent more juice." More than what? Inquiry showed "only that this juicer got that much more juice than an old-fashioned hand-reamer," though it still might be the poorest electrical juicer on the market.

"Twice as many" or "twice as much" means nothing unless you know: More than what?

Psst! I've got a hot stock tip I'll sell you ... Watch out, warns Dr. Simon at the University of Maryland. A stock-picker's great record may be more luck than skill. Statistics tell us that some people, by chance alone, will pick a portfolio that will go up, just as a few coin-flippers among many flip several heads in a row.

Business: Ringing up Retail Sales

Author Huff urges us to consider: "What's missing?"

A business story says that April retail sales are well ahead of those for April the year before. Left unstated: the fact that Easter came in March the first year and in April the second.

Always look for other alternate explanations.

Elections: what is history?

For post-election analysis, political reporters often compare the final results not only to what the polls had predicted, but with historical voting patterns. And that became part of the broader story in the days after the 2004 Bush–Kerry election.

Official election results showed that Bush had won Ohio – and with that the nation. But some controversy simmered over the results in the

Cleveland area, where there were problems with voting machines and long lines.

Some Kerry aides looked at results from the 2000 Gore–Bush presidential election, and said this comparison showed that Kerry had received fewer Cleveland area votes than "predicted." They urged Kerry to seek a recount.

However, top election statisticians tell us it's best to look at historical data over several elections. And that type of analysis showed that Kerry had done *better* than expected in the Cleveland area. Kerry accepted defeat in Ohio without a recount. And the important thing for the history books now is that Bush again took his oath of office in January 2005.[14]

Don't base your reporting solely on what an advocate tells you.

World affairs: confusing counts

Professor I. Richard Savage, at Yale University, notes that news of the Vietnam War "gave ample suggestion that statistics was being used for self-deception." He quotes then Defense Secretary Robert McNamara: "You couldn't reconcile the number of the enemy, the level of infiltration, the body count, and the resulting figures. It just didn't add up. I never did get ... a balanced equation."[15]

Nor did perceptive reporters. Journalists should trust their instincts and ask more questions.

Crime: where you draw the line

Washington, D.C., was dubbed the nation's "murder capital" in the late 1980s, based on statistics from cities across the nation. Malcolm Gladwell, a *Washington Post* financial reporter, used his numbers-sense to show that the label was undeserved. Washington's problem, he found, had more to do with the historical accident that produced that city's political boundaries.[16]

Many other cities encompass relatively large – and relatively safe – suburban fringes. Washington, D.C., is not part of any state and has never been able to annex suburban areas that could dilute the city's crime statistics. If Washington's borders took in "35 percent of the surrounding metro population, as Philadelphia's borders do, the city's murder rate would drop out of the top 10," Gladwell showed.

This isn't just a crime phenomenon. It distorts the Washington, D.C., infant mortality rate too, Gladwell discovered. And other things, no doubt.

Compare cities with care.

DNA: *history and a medical frontier*

The political opponents of Thomas Jefferson, the nation's third president, leveled a charge in 1802 that reverberates to this day. They alleged that Jefferson had fathered a son of one of his slaves, Sally Hemings. Historical speculation simmered for almost two centuries before coming to a boil.

Jefferson is no longer around to give a blood sample, which limits the type of DNA testing that can be done to see whether there is a paternity link. But some enterprising scientists did the next best thing. They tested blood from descendants of Jefferson's paternal grandfather and compared it with blood from Hemings's descendants. The Jefferson and the Hemings descendants both had a male-line DNA marker that would normally be found in less than 1 percent of all men.

"The simplest and most probable explanations for our molecular [DNA] findings are that Thomas Jefferson ... was the father of Eston [Hemings]," the researchers reported in the journal *Nature* in 1998. Then they added: "We cannot completely rule out other explanations of our findings based on illegitimacy in various lines of descent." For example: A male relative of Jefferson might have introduced the genetic marker into the Hemings family tree. But there is no historical evidence to support such conjecture, the researchers added.

Many news publications weren't as cautious as the researchers. The word "proof" was used too often, although some publications did use careful terms such as "found evidence" or "suggests." The Statistical Assessment Service, a watchdog group that tracks news reports, noted that one newspaper went so far as to headline the story: "Adulterer on Mt. Rushmore."[17]

Just to make the scientific caution crystal clear: The head of the research team wrote a letter, published in the *New York Times,* saying again, "This study could not prove anything conclusively."

Just to make the practical point clear: The Thomas Jefferson Memorial Foundation said in early 2000 that, based on both the scientific and the historical evidence, it now accepts the "strong likelihood" that Jefferson fathered at least one Hemings child.[18]

Proper qualifications don't weaken a story; they add credibility.

DNA continues in the news in another important way. Experimental gene therapy has been tried in some patients, and this use of DNA may someday be used to combat a wide variety of diseases. But it must pass the statistical and other tests of science, and overcome concerns raised by serious side effects in some early patients.

Who makes more money? comparing apples with oranges

In the midst of the woes generated by the Great Recession, a number of studies appeared, often from conservative think tanks, claiming that government workers were making more money in salaries and benefits than their counterparts in the private sector. But then the federal Office of Personnel Management struck back. Using data from the Bureau of Labor Statistics, they showed that when we control for level of work and region of the country, the private sector makes more. In an undifferentiated analysis, federal workers seem to make more because so many of them are professionals and managers, and few are the high-school-only-educated waiters and laborers found in the private sector.[19]

Apples should be compared to apples, not to oranges.

Worker safety: hidden numbers

A page-one article in the *New York Times* told us that "workers at New York City building sites have the highest rate of death from unsafe conditions among the nation's 35 largest cities."[20]

How many workers have been dying? We had to read to the 14th paragraph, on the jump page inside the second section, to learn that from 1979 through 1985 the numbers of deaths varied from 7 to 15 a year. We had to get to the 25th paragraph to find the *rate* described in the first paragraph: 7.61 deaths for each billion dollars of construction, much higher than the average 3.3 deaths in the 35 cities.

Why couldn't the story have told us right at the outset: "Between 7 and 15 New York City workers a year die in construction accidents"? Fear of numbers? Fear that even *New York Times* readers fear numbers? Fear that 7 to 15 deaths a year wouldn't sound impressive in the big, violent city? We don't know.

Don't bury the numbers if the numbers are the story.

Entertainment: rocket-car risk

This tale may just be a tale, but it's a fun one that a Harvard biologist (in a letter appearing in the journal *Science*) used to make a point about viewing things from different perspectives:

Back in 1974, Evel Knievel was about to attempt to jump over the Snake River Canyon in a rocket car. The car's designer told a TV reporter that Knievel had about an 80 percent chance of success.

"That good?" replied the TV reporter, apparently coming into the interview fearing the worst.

"Good?" shot back the designer. "You think that's *good*?"

We don't know what Knievel thought of his chances. Was he successful? It depends on how you define success. His rocket car didn't make it across. But an emergency parachute did open to save Knievel's life.

Remember: Risk perception varies from one person to another.

Weather: bedroom and other behavior

We regularly read about weather records – the hottest day, coldest day, or whatever in so many years. One of this book's coauthors (Cope) went to other statistics to tell readers of the Minneapolis–St. Paul *Star Tribune* how the weather really affects their everyday lives.

Do Minnesota's long, cold nights in December and January bring bedroom behavior that results in an increased birth rate nine months later? No. March is the leading month for births in Minnesota. Count back the gestational nine months and you're at June – the month with the shortest nights in the year.

Do traffic fatalities rise in Minnesota during the ice and snow season? No. Total accidents increase. But that's primarily because of fender-benders. Higher speeds in the summer, along with more travel then, explain the higher death toll at that time.

Does it get too cold even for burglars and thieves? Probably. Minneapolis's major crime rates are lowest during winter months.[21]

And even reporters can fudge numbers a bit. When a well-known reporter and columnist applied for his first job out of college, his application stated that he "knew the streets of Paris as well as he knew the streets of Philadelphia." True enough, since he'd never been to either city.[22]

Statistics are serious business, but sometimes you can have fun with them.

Scientific fraud: lessons from Korea

A team of South Korean researchers made big headlines around the world in 2004 and 2005. Dr. Hwang Woo-Suk and colleagues claimed that they had cloned human embryos and extracted stem cells from them. Their reports – first claiming one success, then 11 more – were published by the prestigious journal *Science*.

155

The research was widely portrayed as a huge breakthrough toward realizing the full medical potential of human embryo stem cells, which eventually may be used to treat many diseases. And the Korean report also supported some Americans' concerns that, because of limitations placed on U.S. federal funding of this type of research, other countries would gain a competitive advantage.

By late 2005, the Korean researchers were back in the headlines – with allegations that their research claims were a fraud. Tips from young researchers in Hwang's lab had led to a closer look by a TV investigative news program in Seoul. Then Seoul National University investigated – and fired Hwang. *Science* magazine retracted the articles.[23]

From time to time, there are science-fraud scandals in the United States, although few have been this sensational. Can medical reporters be expected to uncover fraudulent research, when even highly qualified peer reviewers at a leading scientific journal are fooled? No. In fact, American reporters did seek out comments from American experts on the cloning claims, and these experts were quite accepting of the Korean research.

Yet there are lessons for journalists here: The bigger the claim, the more that reporters need to ask probing questions. And, sometimes, some skepticism may be in order.

The Korean case may make journalists think more about the unthinkable subject of scientific fraud. After all, scientists are thinking and writing about it.

Missing Numbers

More numbers could help many news reports. Here are some examples:

Sports stadiums and taxpayers

A *New York Times* article, reporting on a proposed $1-billion-plus city investment in three stadiums, cited an official's estimate that for each dollar invested, taxpayers could expect a return of $3.50 to $4.50 over 30 years.

Daniel Okrent, the *Times'* public editor (ombudsman), pointed out that another number is needed to keep the stadium subsidy in perspective. Thirty-year U.S. Treasury bonds could provide a $4 return per dollar invested – with much more safety of capital.[24]

Courts and punishments

Okrent also cited, in the same column, two examples of court reporting that had missing numbers:

- An article stated that a criminal defendant could face up to 85 years in prison, without mentioning the *likely* sentence.
- Other articles tell of suits against companies for tens to hundreds of millions of dollars. Missing are any specifics that would indicate that the figures are more than the plaintiff attorneys' dreamy hopes.

Autism and kids' shots

Autism tends to appear at the age that toddlers get their vaccine shots. But extensive studies have found no cause-and-effect link between the youngsters' immunizations and autism. A 2004 report by the prestigious Institute of Medicine of the National Academy of Sciences said it's time to move on to genetics and other areas in the search for the cause.[25]

Still, some worried parents won't allow their children to be vaccinated against measles and other dangerous diseases. Some health experts fear this shunning of shots could grow.

In many news reports, the missing numbers are the tolls these childhood diseases took before the vaccines were available. Back then, measles alone killed about 450 American children a year, polio crippled thousands, and rubella was a major cause of birth defects.

Postscript: The British doctor whose research linking vaccines and autism caused public alarm was banned from practicing medicine in the UK. He was found guilty of severe ethical lapses, including receiving funding for his research from lawyers who represented clients suing vaccine makers.[26]

GIGO and the Bottom Line

Robert Samuelson, *Newsweek*'s economics columnist, advises us: "If you are going to use a number, you'd better know where it comes from, how reliable it is and whether it means what it seems to mean." The garbage-in, garbage-out (GIGO) problem has been with us a long time. Or as British economist Sir Josiah Stamp (1880–1941) once put it: "The government [is] very keen on amassing statistics. They collect them, add them, raise them to the *n*th power, take the cube root and prepare wonderful diagrams. But you must never forget that every one of these figures comes in the first instance from the village watchman, who just puts down what he damn well pleases."[27]

Data-gathering is *far* better today. But in this GIGO era, watch out for garbage men.

This book's bottom line:

Much of *News & Numbers* has necessarily dealt with how scientific studies and other statistical claims can go wrong. But as journalists, we must walk the line between being too skeptical, even cynical, and too gullible. Then our readers and viewers will more fully appreciate the true worth of the numbers that make news, as well as their limitations.

Notes

1. Nancy Lyon Spruill, "Perspective: Politics by the Numbers," *Washington Post*, September 20, 1984.
2. "Meat Export Rise Could Buoy Prices," *Washington Post*, March 31, 1973.
3. Daniel Seligman, "We're Drowning in Phony Statistics," *Fortune*, November 1961.
4. Lake Wobegon is a fictional town in Minnesota, presented as the boyhood home of Garrison Keillor, who reports the "News from Lake Wobegon" on the radio show *A Prairie Home Companion*.
5. Anemona Hartocollis, "New Math: No One Is Below Average," *New York Times*, June 20, 1999; and "Liar, Liar, Pants on Fire," *New York Times*, December 12, 1999.
6. Richard Willing, "Police Lineups Encourage Wrong Picks, Experts Say," *USA Today*, November 25, 2002; "Survey of Police Finds Key Advice Is Ignored," *Pittsburgh Post-Gazette*, May 9, 2005; Kate Zernike, "Study Fuels a Growing Debate Over Police Lineups," *New York Times*, April 19, 2006.
7. Carl Bialik, "The Link Between Dinner and Drugs," *Wall Street Journal Online*, October 7, 2005, and other news reports.
8. Rob Stein, "Researchers Look at Prayer and Healing," *Washington Post*, March 24, 2006.
9. Dan Barry, "A New Account of Sep. 11 Loss, with 40 Fewer Souls to Mourn," *New York Times*, October 29, 2003, and other news reports.
10. Julian L. Simon, "Probability—'Batter's Slump' and Other Illusions," *Washington Post*, August 9, 1987.
11. Mosteller, personal communication.
12. Hooke, *How to Tell the Liars*.
13. Huff, *How to Lie*.

14. Various news reports, and talks with statisticians.
15. I. Richard Savage, presidential address, American Statistical Association, Philadelphia, August 14, 1984.
16. Malcolm Gladwell, "Murder Capital We're Not," *Washington Post*, April 16, 1989.
17. This section is based on various news reports about the Thomas Jefferson history case, as well as the scientific report by Eugene Foster et al. in *Nature* 396 (November 5, 1998): 13–14 and 27–28. Foster further discussed the case in a letter to the editor, *New York Times*, November 9, 1998. The press's performance got a drubbing in "Vital Stats: The Numbers Behind the News," the newsletter of the Statistical Assessment Service, November 1998, which noted the headline that we cited.
18. Dennis Cauchon, "Foundation Agrees: Jefferson Probably Fathered Slave's Kids," *USA Today,* front-page in-depth article, January 27, 2000.
19. Lisa Rein, "Fighting Back over Government Salaries," *Washington Post*, August 17, 2010.
20. "Deaths in Building-Site Accidents Found to Be Highest in New York," *New York Times*, September 21, 1987.
21. Lewis Cope, "How the Weather Affects Minnesotans' Lives," *Star Tribune* of Minneapolis–St. Paul, November 5, 1985.
22. Adam Bernstein, "Columnist Explored Public-Policy Issues from Conservative Perspective," *Washington Post*, August 17, 2010.
23. From various news reports. Journalists may be particularly interested in: Gina Kolata, "A Cloning Scandal Rocks a Pillar of Science Publishing, *New York Times*, December 18, 2005; James Brooke, "A Korean TV Show Reports, and the Network Cancels It," *New York Times*, December 21, 2005.
24. Daniel Okrent, "Numbed by the Numbers," *New York Times*, January 23, 2005.
25. Kimberly Pierceall, "Vaccine–Autism Link Is Discounted," *Wall Street Journal*, May 19, 2004, and other news reports.
26. John Burns, "British Medical Council Bars Doctor Who Linked Vaccine with Autism," *New York Times*, May 24, 2010.
27. Robert Samuelson, "The Joy of Statistics," *Newsweek*, November 4, 1985.

Epilogue

The Making of Good Journalists

Shortly before his death, Victor Cohn, the originator and now coauthor of *News & Numbers*, was asked by the Council for the Advancement of Science Writing to jot down his thoughts on what makes a good medical reporter. He did – but quickly added that his thinking applied to all good journalists. So with a few word changes to reflect this broader view:

A good reporter is, first of all, a reporter after a story, not just to cover an assignment or a beat, but a story that's interesting and important.

A good reporter also has fun, fun talking to many fascinating and dedicated people, fun writing copy that zings and captures the reader, fun that injects passion into the job, for it is a job that needs passion.

A good reporter reports for all the people, not for the experts or for the people in the story, not even for editors or news directors.

A good reporter is privileged to contribute to the great fabric of news that democracy requires. There is no more important job than giving people the information they need to work, to survive, to enjoy life, to participate in and maintain a free and democratic society."

News & Numbers: A Writer's Guide to Statistics, Third Edition. Victor Cohn and Lewis Cope with Deborah Cohn Runkle.
© 2012 Victor Cohn and Lewis Cope. Published 2012 by Blackwell Publishing Ltd.

We hope this book will be helpful not only to reporters, but to all journalists and to other communicators as well. This includes all the writers, editors, copy editors, news directors, bloggers, and others who play key roles in our important and rewarding profession.

To all of you: May you find great satisfaction in spreading the words and numbers that allow our society to thrive.

Glossary

absolute survival (or **observed survival**) The actual proportion of a group still living after a certain time. Often compared with relative survival. *See also* **relative survival**.

actuarial method *See* **life table method**.

adjusted rate (or **standardized rate**) A way of comparing two groups that differ in some important variable (e.g., age) by mathematically eliminating the effect of that variable. *See also* **crude rate**.

analytic study An observational study that seeks to analyze or explain the occurrence of a disease or characteristic in a population.

attack rate The incidence of new cases of a disease in a population, often during an epidemic.

background (or **background rate**) The already occurring rate of some physiological effect or physical phenomenon (such as radiation) in a population or locality. This is distinguished from the rate added by some additional influence.

bias The influence of irrelevant or even spurious factors or association on a result or conclusion.

blinding A method of keeping study participants and, if possible, researchers unaware of which participants are in an experimental group (e.g., those getting a new drug) and which are in a control group (those getting an older drug or a placebo). The aim is to prevent people's hopes and expectations from affecting the reported results.

News & Numbers: A Writer's Guide to Statistics, Third Edition. Victor Cohn and Lewis Cope with Deborah Cohn Runkle.
© 2012 Victor Cohn and Lewis Cope. Published 2012 by Blackwell Publishing Ltd.

case–control study A study that compares individuals affected by a disease with a comparable group of people who do not have that disease, to seek possible causes or associations.

chi-square test One commonly used mathematical technique to measure the probability that what is observed didn't occur by chance alone.

clinical trial A research study to determine whether an experimental treatment works, or to see whether there are new ways to use a known treatment. Clinical trials answer questions about the safety and effectiveness of drugs, other treatments, diagnostic procedures, and vaccines. At its best, a clinical trial is a study involving two (or more) comparable, randomly selected groups; for example, an experimental group that gets an experimental drug, and an untreated (or differently treated) control group. *See also* **control group**, **crossover study**, **external controls**, **historical controls**.

cohort study (or **incidence study**) A study of a group of people, or cohort, followed over time to see how some disease or diseases develop.

confidence interval (or **confidence limits**) In an estimate or measurement of a result in a sample, the range within which the truth probably lies.

confounder(s) (or **confounding variables** or **covariables**) Other factors or explanations that may affect a result or conclusion.

control group A comparison group. A group of individuals used by a researcher as a standard for comparison, to see how they differ from an experimental group (such as people receiving a new treatment). *See also* **blinding**.

correlation The extent to which two or more variables in an association are related. *See also* **linear relationship**.

crossover study A clinical trial in which the same patients get two or more treatments in succession, thus acting as their own controls.

crude rate The actual rate of cases of a disease in a population, without adjustment. *See also* **adjusted rate**.

denominator The number or population representing the total universe in which an event might happen.

descriptive study A study that describes the incidence, prevalence, and mortality of a disease in a population.

design The plan or method of a study or experiment.

distribution The summary of a collection of measurements or values showing how the results of a study, for example, fall along a scale.

dose–response relationship The relationship between the dose of some drug or other agent, or the extent of some exposure, and a physiological response. A dose–response effect means that the effect increases with the dose.

ecological fallacy An assumption, based on observing a number of cases in a population, that there is a cause-and-effect relationship that also applies to populations in other locations.

ecological study In epidemiology, a study seeking a relationship between illness and environmental conditions.

epidemiology The study of cases and patterns to seek the causes of health and diseases.

excess risk (or **excess rate**) An increased rate due to some known or unknown cause.

expected rate A rate adjusted to eliminate the effect of age or some other variable. This can be used for comparison with a rate in a similar population subjected to same effect. For example, the lung cancer rate in nonsmokers can be compared to the rate in smokers, adjusted to eliminate age differences in the two groups.

experimental group The treated group in a study, in contrast to an untreated or more conventionally treated control group.

external controls Use of results of other studies (rather than a simultaneously observed control group) to gauge the effects of some treatment.

false negative The failure to find a result or effect when there is one. *Treatment study*: The false indication that a medical treatment is not working when it really is working. *Diagnostic test*: The false indication that a person doesn't have the medical problem when she or he actually does have that problem. A false negative also can be called a Type II error.

false positive Finding a result or effect when it really doesn't exist. *Treatment study*: The false indication that a medical treatment is working when it really is not working. *Diagnostic test*: The false indication that a person has a medical problem when he or she actually doesn't have that problem. A false positive also can be called a Type I error.

Gaussian curve *See* **normal distribution**.

historical controls Comparison of the results in an experimental group with results in former, often old, reports or records.

hypothesis A tentative statement or supposition, which may then be tested through research. *See also* **null hypothesis**.

incidence rate The occurrence of some event, such as the number of individuals who get a disease, divided by a total given population per unit of time.

independent variable In a two-variable relationship, the underlying variable that affects the incidence of the dependent variable. Weather, for example, as it affects the incidence of colds.

individualistic fallacy An assumption that the results in a small and unrepresentative number of cases also apply to a larger population.

interquartile range The interval between the 75th and 25th percentiles in a data set. This is the middle 50 percent of a distribution, avoiding the extreme values at either end.

intervention study An epidemiological study in which there is some intervention in some subjects to modify a supposed cause of disease.

inverse relationship A negative correlation between two variables. The way that one increases as the other decreases. *Example*: a runner's average speed goes down as his or her weight goes up.

life table method (or **actuarial method**) In a five-year study of cancer, for example, a way of predicting the final result although some of the subjects began treatment less than five years earlier. The conclusion is based on experience to date with some participants in the study and reasonable expectation for the others.

linear relationship A positive (or negative) correlation between two variables, showing up as a straight, steadily rising (or falling) set of data points on a graph.

mean The arithmetic average. The sum of all the values divided by the number of values.

median The value or number that divides a population into equal halves.

meta-analysis A way of combining the results of several studies to draw conclusions.

mode The most frequently occurring value in a distribution.

morbidity rate The incidence of a particular disease or, often, all illnesses per unit of time (often per year) in a population.

mortality rate The incidence of deaths per unit of time, most often per year, in a population.

multivariate analysis A way of studying many variables to try to understand the relationships between them. For example, a way of relating many variables in a study to find those that are truly important.

166

natural experiment An experiment of nature or a change in human habits that can be studied to draw valuable conclusions.

nonparametric method A technique of examining data that does not rely on a numerical distribution. For example, using a plus or minus sign rather than a count to record a result.

normal distribution A collection of individual values that show up in a graph as a bell-shaped (or Gaussian) curve, high in the middle and low at each end. To the layman, and in common use, anything approximating this form. To a mathematician, a curve complying with a more precise formula.

null hypothesis A way an investigator can scrupulously test an initial, hopeful hypothesis. The researcher hypothesizes that a treatment, for example, has no effect, then sees if the results disprove this negative assumption.

observational study A study that simply observes and describes, offering clues but not a positive determination of cause and effect. *Example*: the simultaneous occurrence of acid rain and the losses in plant and animal life.

observed rate The actual rate of a disease or condition, without adjustment to eliminate the effect of age or other variables.

parallel study A clinical study comparing two similar groups simultaneously given different treatments or treatment versus no treatment.

parameter As most commonly used, a measurable characteristic or property.

peer review Evaluation of a medical or scientific report or proposal by other qualified people.

placebo A supposedly ineffective pill or agent used in a control group to gauge the effect of an actual treatment in another group. Experimenters often must allow for a placebo effect, a response caused by suggestion.

population In statistics, any group or collection of relevant units – people, events, objects, test scores, physiologic values, or whatever – from which a sample may be drawn for study.

power In statistics, the probability of finding an effect if one is in fact present, dependent on adequate size of the sample or population studied.

prevalence rate The total case rate of a disease or condition in a given population at a given time. In epidemiology, a prevalence (or current or cross-sectional) study examines the relationship between a disease and other variables in a population at a particular time.

probability A calculation of what may be expected, based on what has happened in the past under similar conditions.

prospective study A study of morbidity and mortality and other characteristics in a group while it is under study. By comparison, a retrospective study examines a group exposed in the past. Prospective studies watch diseases develop; retrospective studies look at people who already have a disease.

protocol The plan and rules for a study, set prior to its implementation. The protocol includes, among other things, who may participate in the study, the dosages of drugs to be used and tests to be conducted, and the duration of the study.

***P* value** (or **probability value**) The probability that an observed result or effect could have occurred by chance if there had actually been no real effect.

randomization Division of a sample into two or more comparable groups by some random method that eliminates biased selection.

random variation (or **chance**) The way a coin will successively turn up heads or tails if flipped in just the same way.

range A measure of spread; for example, the spread between the highest and lowest values in a distribution.

rate The proportion of some disease or condition in a group per unit of time, with a numerator and denominator (stated or implied) telling us "so many per so many per year or other unit of time."

regression (or **regression analysis**) A mathematical method commonly used to determine how greatly various other or independent variables affect a dependent variable or outcome.

regression toward the mean The tendency for an unusually high or low value at one time to be less extreme at a second measurement.

relative risk (or **risk ratio**) A comparison of two morbidity or mortality rates by calculating the ratio of one to the other.

relative survival This is a mathematically produced (in statistical parlance, adjusted) figure that is calculated to show the chance of survival from one disease alone (commonly cancer), rather than survival from the many diseases and causes that always affect a population. Relative survival thus appears longer, as a rule, than actual (known as absolute or observed) survival.

reliability The reproducibility of a result when a test or experiment is repeated.

retrospective study *See* **prospective study**.

risk assessment A quantitative estimate of the degree of hazard to a population presented by some agent or technology or decision. A risk–benefit assessment attempts to weigh possible risks against possible benefits.

sample A part of a population, selected by a technique called sampling, to represent the whole population.

self-controlled study A clinical study in which the subjects (participants) act as their own controls, with the researcher comparing periods of treatment with periods of either no treatment or some other treatment.

sensitivity/specificity *Sensitivity* is the ability of a test to avoid false negatives; its ability to identify a disease or condition in those who have it. *Specificity* is a test's ability to avoid mistaken identifications – that is, false positives.

significance In an experiment or clinical trial, statistical significance means there is only a small statistical probability that the same result could have been found by chance alone.

specificity *See* **sensitivity/specificity**.

spread, measurement of *See* **range**.

statistics As a scientific discipline or method, a way of gathering and analyzing data to extract information, seek causation, and calculate probabilities.

stratification Separation of a sample or population into subgroups, according to some characteristic.

strength Statistically, the strength of an association. The greater the odds of an effect, the stronger the association.

survival *See* **absolute survival, relative survival**.

Type I error *See* **false positive**.

Type II error *See* **false negative**.

universe A population. The whole group of people or units under consideration.

validity The truth or accuracy of a statistic or an experimental result or conclusion.

variability (or **variation**) Fluctuation from measurement to measurement, common in all measurement.

variable Any factor, measurement, characteristic, or event that can vary – and, in a study or experiment, can affect the outcome.

vital statistics The systematically collected statistics on births, deaths, marriages, divorces, and other life events. More broadly, the statistics of life, health, disease, and death. In particular, the statistics that measure progress, or lack of it, against disease.

Bibliography

Statistics Texts and Manuals

Freedman, David, Robert Pisani, and Roger Purves. *Statistics* (New York: W. W. Norton, 1978). A complete, readable, and even entertaining statistics text, with many examples and anecdotes and a conversational style.

Leaverton, Paul F. *A Review of Biostatistics: A Program for Self-Instruction*, 2nd edn. (Boston: Little, Brown, 1978). A course of instruction in 87 concise pages.

Moore, David S. *Statistics: Concepts and Controversies*, 2nd edn. (New York: W. H. Freeman, 1986). A full-size work that lives up to its blurb: "the heart of statistics with careful explanations and real-life examples, avoiding unnecessarily complicated mathematics."

Moses, Lincoln. *Think and Explain with Statistics* (Reading, Mass.: Addison-Wesley, 1986). By a Stanford professor and one of American statistics' major figures. A popular statistics text that is strong on practical use of statistics.

White, David M., and Seymour Levine. *Elementary Statistics for Journalists* (New York: Macmillan, 1954). Professor Michael Greenberg at Rutgers calls this "the best introduction for journalists who have no background nor any time to take a course."

Youden, W. J. *Experimentation and Measurement* (Washington, D.C.: U.S. Government Printing Office, 1984). We recommend this as a supplemental source. Written by a consultant to the National Bureau of Standards (now National Institute of Standards and Technology), it focuses on use of statistics in measurement but also has many valuable sections of statistics in general.

Zeisel, Hans. *Say It with Figures*, 6th edn. (New York: Harper and Row, 1985). Both a text and a guide to understanding – and questioning – social statistics.

News & Numbers: A Writer's Guide to Statistics, Third Edition. Victor Cohn and Lewis Cope with Deborah Cohn Runkle.
© 2012 Victor Cohn and Lewis Cope. Published 2012 by Blackwell Publishing Ltd.

Epidemiology Texts – In Fact,
Simple Statistics Courses

Friedman, Gary D. *Primer of Epidemiology*, 3rd edn. (New York: McGraw-Hill, 1987). A Kaiser epidemiologist and biostatistician, Friedman covers much of statistics, with examples from medicine and epidemiology. A treasure, concise and easy to read and follow.

Lillienfeld, Abraham, and David E. Lillienfeld. *Foundations of Epidemiology*, 2nd edn. (New York: Oxford University Press, 1980). A standard, for good reason.

On the Statistics of Real-Life
Situations – Good-Reading Companions to Texts

Campbell, Stephen K. *Flaws and Fallacies in Statistical Thinking* (Englewood Cliffs, N.J.: Prentice-Hall, 1974). The emphasis is on recognizing statistical frauds and whoppers, intentional or otherwise, and distinguishing between valid and faulty reasoning.

Huff, Darrell. *How to Live with Statistics* (New York: W. W. Norton, 1954). Short, provocative, amusing.

Tanur, Judith M., ed., and by Frederick Mosteller, William H. Kruskal, Erich L. Lehmann, Richard F. Link, Richard S. Pieters, and Gerald R. Rising. *Statistics: A Guide to the Unknown*, 3rd edn. (Pacific Grove, Calif.: Wadsworth and Brooks-Cole, 1989). An anomaly, a good work produced by a committee. A series of chapters on the practical applications of almost every branch of statistics, from surveys to medical experiments to weather to sports.

Vogt, Thomas M. *Making Health Decisions: An Epidemiologic Perspective on Staying Well* (Chicago: Nelson-Hall, 1983). For the general reader or the journalist, guidance and good reading on "making sound judgments about claims and counter-claims" about health and disease.

Weaver, Warren. *Lady Luck: The Theory of Probability* (Garden City, N.Y.: Doubleday Anchor Books, 1963). All you want to know about probability, from the amusingly anecdotal to the technical.

On Applying Statistics
and Polling Methods to Reporting

Meyer, Philip. *Precision Journalism: A Reporter's Introduction to Social Science Methods*, 2nd edn. (Bloomington: Indiana University Press, 1979). The first and now classic work in this area, by a longtime *Detroit Free Press* and Knight reporter and editor, who became a professor at the University of North Carolina, Chapel Hill.

On Statistics in Medicine, Biomedical Research, and Clinical Trials

Written for Researchers and Physicians, but with Much Rich Detail for Conscientious Medical Reporters

Bailar, John C., III, and Frederick Mosteller, eds. *Medical Uses of Statistics* (Waltham, Mass.: NEJM Books, 1986). This grew out of a series in the *New England Journal of Medicine*.

Ingelfinger, J. A., Frederick Mosteller, L. A. Thibodeau, and J. H. Ware. *Biostatistics in Clinical Medicine*, 2nd edn. (New York: Macmillan, 1986).

Shapiro, Stanley H., and Thomas A. Louis, eds. *Clinical Trials: Issues and Approaches* (New York: Marcel Dekker, 1983).

Warren, Kenneth S. *Coping with the Biomedical Literature: A Primer for the Scientists and the Clinician* (New York: Praeger, 1981).

On Health Hazards

Legator, Marvin S., Barbara L. Harper, and Michael J. Scott, eds. *The Health Detective's Handbook: A Guide to the Investigation of Environmental Health Hazards by Nonprofessionals* (Baltimore, Maryland: Johns Hopkins University Press, 1985). A marvelous practical guide for concerned citizens and inquiring reporters.

Related Publications by Victor Cohn, Coauthor of this Book

Cohn, Victor. *Reporting on Risk: Getting it Right in an Age of Risk* (Washington, D.C.: The Media Institute, 1990). A book about environmental and related risk reporting, which expands on the environmental chapter in *News & Numbers*.

Cohn, Victor. *A Newsperson's Guide to Reporting Health Plan Performance*. A booklet prepared independently by Cohn and distributed by the American Association of Health Plans, Washington, D.C. (published in 2000).

Index

References to notes are entered as, for example, 7n.

News & Numbers: A Writer's Guide to Statistics, Third Edition. Victor Cohn and
Lewis Cope with Deborah Cohn Runkle.
© 2012 Victor Cohn and Lewis Cope. Published 2012 by Blackwell Publishing Ltd.

Printed and bound by: Sheridan Group
UK Ltd
BR35/1

Printed and bound by CPI Group (UK) Ltd, Croydon, CR0 4YY

27/10/2024

14580369-0001